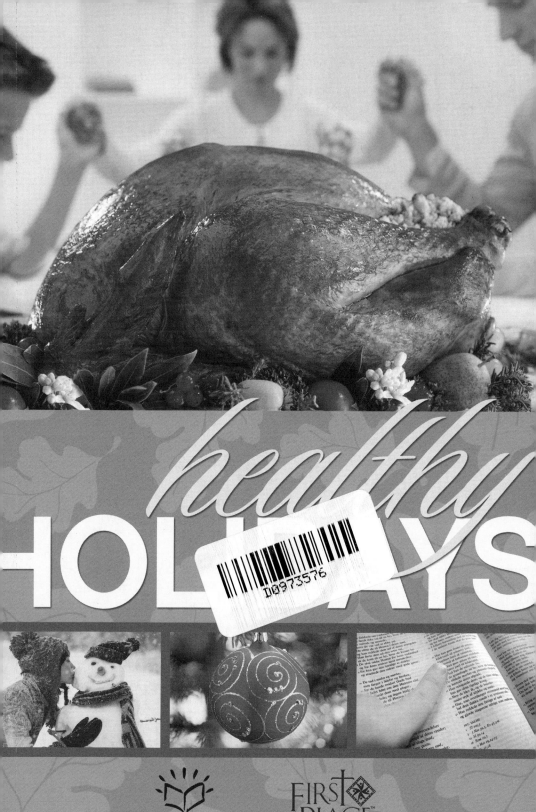

healthy
HOLIDAYS

Gospel Light

FIRST PLACE

Gospel Light

Gospel Light is a Christian publisher dedicated to serving the local church. We believe God's vision for Gospel Light is to provide church leaders with biblical, user-friendly materials that will help them evangelize, disciple and minister to children, youth and families.

It is our prayer that this Gospel Light resource will help you discover biblical truth for your own life and help you minister to others. May God richly bless you.

For a free catalog of resources from Gospel Light, please contact your Christian supplier or contact us at 1-800-4-GOSPEL or www.gospellight.com.

PUBLISHING STAFF
William T. Greig, Chairman • **Dr. Elmer L. Towns,** Senior Consulting Publisher
• **Bayard Taylor, M.Div.,** Senior Editor, Biblical and Theological Issues

ISBN 0-8307-3374-4
© 2005 First Place
All rights reserved.
Printed in the U.S.A.

CAUTION
The information contained in this book is intended to be solely informational and educational. It is assumed that the First Place participant will consult a medical or health professional before beginning this or any other weight-loss or physical fitness program.

Contents

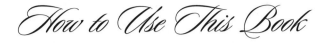

How to Use This Book

But seek first his kingdom and his righteousness,
and all these things will be given to you as well.
MATTHEW 6:33

This book is not the typical First Place Bible study. This is a special tool to help you stay on course through the holidays. The holidays can be very busy with many social events, shopping expeditions and church activities. This book was written to provide order in the hectic holiday season without being a burden on your time. Use this book as a devotional, journal or workbook. It will give you inspiration for each day and also challenge you to stay on course by daily applying the truths presented.

DAILY DEVOTIONAL

One Scripture verse is featured for an entire week. Each daily devotional uses that verse as the reference. The devotionals are holiday related and give insight and encouragement to maintain balance during the holidays.

JOURNAL

Each devotional has a prayer and a journal suggestion. A journal page has been provided for each day to write out your prayers, thoughts and questions.

SMALL GROUPS

You may use this book on your own or in a small-group setting. For more information on how to implement and lead a small group, see the Leader's Guide section at the back of this book. This section has some key features that will be useful and beneficial to your First Place journey.

HOLIDAY HELPS—WELLNESS WORKSHEETS

These worksheets are designed to be interactive and may be completed individually or with a small group. They contain helpful information in the spiritual, emotional, physical and mental areas of your life.

MENUS AND RECIPES

We have provided menus and recipes for a 1,400-calorie Thanksgiving, Christmas and New Year's Day. Recipes for additional holiday favorites are included with the menus.

COMMITMENT RECORDS

To maintain a healthy lifestyle throughout the holidays, Commitment Records have been provided for each week.

To get the most from this book, read a devotional daily, using the journal pages to write your prayers, thoughts and questions. Commit to applying the Holiday Helps that fit your personal needs and interests. Spread some healthy holiday cheer by preparing and sharing the menus and recipes with your friends and family. May the next six weeks take you on a joyful journey toward complete wholeness and health! Here's to the journey!

Gates of Thanksgiving

PRECIOUS MOMENTS

Enter his gates with thanksgiving and his courts with praise;
give thanks to him and praise his name.
PSALM 100:4

Thanksgiving 2001 is indelibly imprinted on my mind forever. That was the day our middle child, Shari, left this earth to spend eternity with Jesus. What could I be thankful for in this devastating loss?

Could I be thankful that an 18-year-old girl chose to drive drunk that fateful night? Could I be thankful that my son-in-law, Jeff, no longer has his wife, or thankful that Shari's three girls, Cara, Christen and Amanda, will grow up without their mom? No, I could never be thankful for any of these circumstances, but there are facets to each of these statements for which I can and do give thanks. In tomorrow's devotional I will share how I have been able to discover things to be thankful for in and through this tragic loss of our daughter.

The following are some reasons for which I am personally thankful to God:

I had the privilege of having Shari in my First Place class when she died. Shari lived 50 miles away from our class location and chose to drive that distance each week to be in my class, which gave me the opportunity to see her every week.

I watched with pride as Shari drove an additional 50 miles each Tuesday to pick up Cheri Lasiter, a lady in our class who has cerebral palsy. When Shari heard that Cheri was paying a huge amount to hire a taxi each week, she insisted on picking her up and keeping her all day. I am filled with pride and thankfulness that Shari was my daughter. I am also very thankful that God had given Shari the gift of mercy so that she empathized with anyone who had a need.

I am most thankful that God allowed me to spend the last day of Shari's life with her. This probably would not have been the case had it not been a holiday or someone's birthday. Since Shari and I were both in First Place, she had brought a sugar-free pumpkin pie for the two of us for dessert. My last memory of Shari was her putting the finishing touches on my Christmas tree before she left our home.

Carole Lewis

Day One

Write about a loss or something painful in your own life, and journal some events surrounding the ordeal for which you can give thanks to God.

Thank You, God, that even when we suffer pain and loss there is always reason to give thanks because of You.

_____

_____

_____

_____

_____

_____

_____

_____

_____

_____

_____

_____

_____

_____

_____

_____

_____

_____

_____

_____

_____

_____

*Enter his gates with thanksgiving and his courts with praise;
give thanks to him and praise his name.*
PSALM 100:4

Gates of Thanksgiving

GOD'S GOODNESS

Enter his gates with thanksgiving and his courts with praise;
give thanks to him and praise his name.
PSALM 100:4

There is always something about God's goodness for which we can give thanks and praise His name. The following are additional reasons for which I choose to be thankful in the midst of the sadness and grief over the death of our daughter, Shari:

Lisa Marie DeLeon, the girl whose car struck Shari, has the opportunity to find Christ through this horrible tragedy. We are working with the victim's assistance program in our state to make contact with her. The man who will work with our family is a minister, and he will share Christ with Lisa Marie. The chaplain at the prison unit where she is incarcerated is also a Christian, and he will be available to teach and mentor her after she finds Christ. I am thankful that if Lisa Marie makes the choice to follow Christ, there is a very real possibility that her entire family will become Christians and the chain of alcoholism will be broken.

The night of Shari's death Jeff told me, "I feel as if I've been in training for this job for the last 20 years." Jeff has always been very involved in the lives of his daughters, because of this he could assume the role of both mother and father to them. I am thankful that God gave my precious daughter a husband like Jeff so that her children have a daddy who shows them by his actions the characteristics of our God.

Cara was 19, Christen was 15, and Amanda was 13 the night their mom was killed. Being forced to grow up without their mom is a real tragedy. I can be thankful that Shari's love will continue in their lives. I can also be thankful that God will be their source of strength because they all know Him personally.

God sent a wonderful young Christian man into Cara's life the year after her mom died. We are so thankful that through the friendship that developed, they fell in love and were married January 8, 2005.

Christen is 18 and back in school. Amanda is 16 and in tenth grade; she is raising a goat through Future Farmers of America that took second place in a show.

How thankful we are that God doesn't forget about us when we suffer, but wraps His loving arms around us and brings healing to our broken hearts.

Carole Lewis

Write about a painful situation. Begin to look for blessings in your situation and thank God for them, and He will come into it and heal your pain.

Dear God, Help me never cease to praise and thank You, for I know that You inhabit the praises of Your children.

_____

_____

_____

_____

_____

_____

_____

_____

_____

_____

_____

_____

_____

_____

_____

_____

_____

_____

Enter his gates with thanksgiving and his courts with praise;
give thanks to him and praise his name.
PSALM 100:4

Gates of Thanksgiving

DINING WITH GOD

Enter his gates with thanksgiving and his courts with praise;
give thanks to him and praise his name.
PSALM 100:4

"I never eat when I can dine," the late Maurice Chevalier once said. This statement made a great impact on me as I was losing 147½ pounds through First Place. I am often asked, "Do you remember how it felt to weigh almost 300 pounds?" The answer is a resounding yes!

I will never forget the physical burden I carried all those years. Much more, I vividly remember the tremendous emotional burden. To this day, when I go out to eat in a restaurant, I remember how it felt when the waiter would escort me to a booth rather than a table. A booth to a large person can be so humiliating and at times virtually impossible to fit into. You always look to see if the table is bolted to the floor because you know the table will have to move to allow you to sit. I preferred to go to the drive-through rather than to dine-in. Maurice hit the nail on the head for me: You definitely eat going through the drive-through, but if you take the time to go into the restaurant, you sit down and dine.

So many of us with weight problems avoid entering in to God's gates for very much the same reasons. I can well remember standing on the outside looking in; but because of being so large, I felt unworthy to enter in to His gates. I felt I had nothing to be thankful for until I lost weight. I came to the reality that I was missing the true blessing of entering in and dining with God. One nice thing about entering in to God's gates is that His gates are "one size fits all." There are no humiliating booths.

God would love for you to enter in to His place of worship this Thanksgiving season and dine with Him. Don't cheat yourself out of a blessing by going through the drive-through to eat. Regardless of your weight on this very day, enter in to His gates and be thankful that God loves you just the way you are.

"I never eat when I can dine." There is a big difference between merely eating and purposely sitting down to dine. Enter in and enjoy your dining experience with God.

Beverly Henson

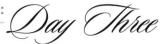
Write about how it would make you feel to actually sit and dine with God. What would you say to Him? How would you feel?

Thank You, Father, for those glorious gates You have provided just for me to enter in. Thank You for loving me just as I am today and for inviting me to dine with You.

_____

_____

_____

_____

_____

_____

_____

_____

_____

_____

_____

_____

_____

_____

_____

_____

_____

_____

_____

*Enter his gates with thanksgiving and his courts with praise;
give thanks to him and praise his name.*
PSALM 100:4

Gates of Thanksgiving

HANDS OF GOD

Enter his gates with thanksgiving and his courts with praise;
give thanks to him and praise his name.
PSALM 100:4

Thanksgiving is a special time of year to focus on God and His goodness. In recent years our family's thoughts go back to Thanksgiving 1997 when my husband, Joe, had a major heart attack. Joe was barely 50 years old and had recently undergone a complete physical. The doctor commented that he would never have to worry about a heart attack.

Two days after Thanksgiving we arrived at our small local hospital thinking that Joe had the flu. Less than an hour later he was in a helicopter on his way to a larger hospital. The doctors took him into what they believed would be a 90-minute surgery to insert a stent, and more than five hours later the doctor returned with bad news. His exact words were, "This has been a nightmare, and I do not think he will make it through the night."

I was allowed to stay at Joe's bedside, and at 3:00 A.M. while staring at him and holding his hand, I was overcome with hopelessness. I told God that I had never even thought of living without those hands, and I could not bear to do so. At that moment our daughter came to the door and said, "Mama, I know you asked me to take all the calls, but this lady says that God asked her to give you a message." It was Emily, from my First Place class, who said, "Kay, I did not hear about Joe until 9:00 tonight. I prayed for an hour and then went to bed." She continued, "A few minutes ago God woke me up, and I knew I was to pray more. I prayed and then started reading the Psalms. While reading Psalm 95, I felt God tell me to call you and read it to you. I argued that it was 3:00 A.M. and the crisis was probably over, plus I didn't know what hospital you were at, but the instructions persisted."

She read Psalm 95 and when she got to verses 3 through 5, I knew exactly what God's message to me was. At the very moment I was staring at Joe's hand feeling hopeless, God decided to send a message to me. First, He needed a faithful servant who could overcome the fear of looking foolish, and who wouldn't think that a wake-up call at 2:30 a.m. was indigestion. He called on Emily, and she overcame her fear enough to tell Sandy that this call was too important to follow my directions. I walked back to Joe's room with the words of a chorus going through my mind: "Do I love you, Lord? Do I love You with all of my heart? Can I trust You, Lord? Can I trust you to do your part?"[1]

I knew God was telling me to take my eyes off Joe's hands and focus on His hands. Joe experienced a terrible crisis just as I returned to his room. All kinds of alarms were going off and the room quickly filled with doctors and nurses. I stood there with such strength after being reminded that God was not only there, He also was in charge of this situation. His words had reminded me that His hands were big enough to gently take Joe to heaven that night if He chose, and that His hands were so big He would not have to set me aside in order to do so. After the crisis Joe took a turn for the better and completely recovered.

I praise God that His hands are bigger than any situation we will face. I thank God today for faithful friends who point me to His Word in time of need.

Kay Smith

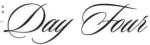
Make a list today of some of your favorite Scripture passages that God has used to comfort or to strengthen you. Make a note of someone with whom you could share one of these passages, letting that person know you have prayed these Scriptures for him or her.

Heavenly Father, I do enter Your gates with thanksgiving and Your courts with praise; I give You thanks today and I praise Your holy name.

_____

_____

_____

_____

_____

_____

_____

_____

_____

_____

_____

_____

_____

_____

_____

_____

_____

_____

_____

_____

Enter his gates with thanksgiving and his courts with praise;
give thanks to him and praise his name.
PSALM 100:4

Gates of Thanksgiving

JOYFUL SONGS

Enter his gates with thanksgiving and his courts with praise;
give thanks to him and praise his name.
PSALM 100:4

The light on my phone was blinking, so I dialed my voice mail to see who had called. Joyful songs rang out in my ear as I listened to my grandchildren sing one of the Scripture memory songs from our First Place Scripture Memory CDs. I called all of my coworkers to come and hear them sing, then saved it on my phone so I could listen to it over and over.

In the *King James Version*, the first verse of Psalm 100 says "Make a joyful noise unto the LORD." Some of us can only make a joyful noise when we sing, but since it thrilled my heart to hear my grandchildren singing to me, I can only imagine how it thrills the heart of God to hear the voices of His children singing praises to Him. Can't you just imagine Him calling to His angels saying, "Come here and listen to My children singing to Me?"

In the church in which I grew up, there was a lady in our choir who was tone deaf and sang the same note on every word of every song. She loved to sing and never missed an opportunity to make a "joyful noise unto the LORD." Even though she never sang in the right key, she sang her heart out to the Lord.

Psalm 100:2 says to "worship the LORD with gladness; come before him with joyful songs." I watch a TV program on Sunday night in which the congregation sings all the old hymns I love. They are singing joyful songs well enough, but when the camera pans the audience, their faces are solemn as they focus on the hymnal, intent on singing every word and hitting every note just right. Not exactly a picture of singing "joyful songs."

God loves to hear His children sing joyful songs to Him. He wants us to lift our faces to Him and sing to Him with joy in our hearts and smiles on our faces. It's okay with Him if we don't get all the words right or if we sing off-key now and then. He just wants us to worship Him with gladness and joyful praise in our hearts.

We have much to be thankful for. Let God know how thankful you are by singing joyful songs to Him this Thanksgiving season.

Pat Lewis

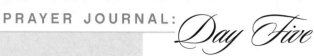
Write a joyful song to the Lord, or write the words of your favorite joyful hymn or chorus in your journal and sing it to Him during your quiet time.

Thank You, Lord, that You gave us a voice to sing joyful songs to You. Let us have a song in our hearts and on our lips this Thanksgiving season as we enter in to Your presence with thanksgiving and praise.

_____

_____

_____

_____

_____

_____

_____

_____

_____

_____

_____

_____

_____

_____

_____

_____

_____

Enter his gates with thanksgiving and his courts with praise;
give thanks to him and praise his name.
PSALM 100:4

Gates of Thanksgiving

JOY IN HIS PRESENCE

Enter his gates with thanksgiving and his courts with praise;
give thanks to him and praise his name.
PSALM 100:4

Shooter is a beautiful black Labrador retriever that our family adopted a couple of years ago. He adores us, and when we arrive home each day, he jumps for joy to just be in our presence. He runs in circles as fast as he can to show us his excitement. If we are seated, he will come over and sit as close as possible without actually getting in our lap. He then proceeds to set his head on the arm of the chair and stare up at us longingly with his big brown eyes. He just wants to be close to us and, with steady determination, will sit at our feet until we give him attention of any kind. He is not picky; he is grateful for a simple pat on the head or a kind word. The more attention I give him, the more he wants and the closer he moves toward me. When Shooter wants to go outside, he runs to the back door and jumps up and down and squeals with anticipation as we turn the doorknob. Once out the door he automatically turns around to see if I will be coming out to play with him. How could you resist those brown eyes looking up at you and a tail wagging like an arm motioning to you to come join him? What an expression of entering gates with thanksgiving and praise!

Through observing Shooter, I am learning how to truly enter God's presence each day with praise and thanksgiving. When the psalmist entered into God's presence he did it with thanksgiving and praise. In the first couple of verses of Psalm 100 the psalmist exhorts us to shout joyfully to the Lord and to serve Him with gladness. Shooter has shown me the importance of beginning my day with joyful anticipation of spending time with the Lord. Our dog doesn't complain that he has been alone for the last 12 hours, that no one has paid him any attention or that he is hungry. He is just thrilled to know we are home. Now, instead of entering my prayer time with the Lord with requests, I take time to praise Him for who He is and thank Him for what He has done. I am learning to express thanks, not just at Thanksgiving, but each day as my eyes open to a new day in His presence. I want to sit at His feet, looking up at Him longingly with thoughts of thankfulness already on my mind. I will be ready with a word of praise on my lips to give to Him as He speaks words of encouragement and hope over me. As He strokes my heart with His truth I will edge closer and closer to Him, enjoying intimacy with my Master. I must thank Shooter for showing me the way to enter into God's presence with praise and thanksgiving. I'll be sure and give him a special treat this Thanksgiving!

Nancy Taylor

Do you enter your daily devotion times with the Lord in an attitude of praise? To help you develop a praiseful attitude, write out a prayer to the Lord praising Him for who He is, listing all His attributes that you can recall and being thankful that He is at home with you!

Lord, forgive me for not entering Your presence each day with praise and thanksgiving. Lord, give me a heart of praise so that my lips will offer praise before making any requests.

_____

_____

_____

_____

_____

_____

_____

_____

_____

_____

_____

_____

_____

_____

_____

_____

_____

_____

Enter his gates with thanksgiving and his courts with praise;
give thanks to him and praise his name.
PSALM 100:4

Gates of Thanksgiving

HAPPY PUPPY, HAPPY PEOPLE

Enter his gates with thanksgiving and his courts with praise;
give thanks to him and praise his name.
PSALM 100:4

I hung up the phone feeling a little sad. Wow! What a good home that would have been for one of our puppies. I was sad because the last puppy had been sold just the evening before to a young couple that lived in an apartment and didn't seem to know a lot about dogs. I was reluctant to make the sale, but when I saw the cash, I gave in. The lady on the phone lived in the country and had owned yellow Labs for years. I thought this would have been such a wonderful home for any puppy. She gave me her number just in case I heard of another litter or had more puppies in the future.

About 10 minutes later, the phone rang and it was the young woman who had bought the last puppy the evening before. She said, "We have a problem; the puppy has not acted happy since we left your house." She said, "We let it ride on the dash of our SUV all the way home, but it didn't eat much dinner. And then we put it in a box and it cried all night; then we found out that our apartment has a no-pets rule." She added that she thought the puppy might be sick.

I laughed and told her that he probably was a little homesick for his family and a little carsick from the ride on the dashboard of their car. She sounded near tears when I interrupted and asked, "Would you like to bring the puppy back?"

She was silent; then in a quiet voice she asked, "You will take the puppy back and refund our money?"

I answered that we would be more than happy to do so.

I was elated because I believed this small puppy was in for a wonderful home in the country. I called the lady seeking a new puppy and gave her the good news. She was happy; I was happy; the young couple were happy, and even the puppy seemed happy when he came bouncing back through our front door. Later I sat at my desk with a smile on my face saying, "Thank You, Lord!"

I thought about that set of events as I read Psalm 100:4. The thought came to me how easy it is to be thankful when we can see a good outcome. But at the same moment I heard that still, small voice say, "That is the kind of thankfulness I am asking you to have in *all* circumstances." Circumstances began to pop into my mind: financial challenges, a family member who has battled alcoholism for 20 years; aging parents with many health challenges; concerns about our two grown kids and grandchildren; the list could go on and on. I realized that it is very easy for me to be thankful and to trust God when circumstances are positive or when I have seen a good outcome. Are we also to be thankful even when we do not see a way out or when circumstances are only getting worse? God's Word says yes.

I have been reminded today to enter into my quiet time with thanksgiving. I will offer up to Him praise for who He is and thankfulness for what He has done. "Be joyful always; pray continually; give thanks in all circumstances, for this is God's will for you in Christ Jesus" (1 Thessalonians 5:16-18).

Kay Smith

Make a list today of the things in your life for which you find it very hard to be thankful. Spend time praying about this, asking God to show you areas of your life or circustances for which you are not thankful.

Heavenly Father, I do enter Your gates with thanksgiving and Your courts with praise; I give You thanks today and I praise Your holy name.

_____

_____

_____

_____

_____

_____

_____

_____

_____

_____

_____

_____

_____

_____

_____

_____

_____

_____

_____

Enter his gates with thanksgiving and his courts with praise; give thanks to him and praise his name.
PSALM 100:4

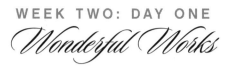

Wonderful Works

OUR PERSONAL MINDER

I praise you because I am fearfully and wonderfully made;
your works are wonderful, I know that full well.
PSALM 139:14

As my family gathers at Thanksgiving to give thanks and praise to our God, we all have special memories of wonderful works the Lord has done for us.

I am reminded of a wonderful work God did in our family when he healed the broken neck of our 14-year-old son. One day while Tim was in the hospital awaiting a very delicate surgery to repair the vertebrae in his neck, Joy Stephens, our pastor's wife, was sitting at his bedside and said, "Tim, the Bible says that you are fearfully and wonderfully made," to which he responded, "Mrs. Stephens, right now I am fearfully," expressing the emotions of everyone.

When the surgery was completed, the doctor said it was a textbook surgery and told the staff assisting him, "There must be someone praying for this young man." Those same people who were praying also gave thanks and praise to God for His wonderful works in saving a young boy's life.

Another more recent wonderful work occurred when God healed a raging infection in the foot of my son, Terry. After removing all of his toes and a portion of his foot, the doctors said they would need to remove his leg up to his knee and possibly higher. They scheduled surgery and we scheduled prayer. God once again did a wonderful work and saved the remainder of Terry's foot and leg.

"When I consider your heavens, the work of your fingers, . . . what is man that you are mindful of him, the son of man that you care for him?" (Psalm 8:3-4). I am fascinated by the term "minders" used in the recent war in Afghanistan and Iraq. Minders are assigned to journalists to watch over the reports they write about the events during the war. The psalmist says God is mindful of us (see Psalm 115:12, *KJV*). He is our personal *minder*, observant and attentive to our every need—always watching over us to perform His wonderful works in our lives.

Pat Lewis

Think of a wonderful work God has done for you or someone you know. Write a prayer of thanksgiving to Him.

Almighty God, Your works are wonderful; we know that full well. You have proven yourself to be faithful in every circumstance, and we give thanks and praise to Your holy and excellent name.

_____

_____

_____

_____

_____

_____

_____

_____

_____

_____

_____

_____

_____

_____

_____

_____

_____

_____

_____

I praise you because I am fearfully and wonderfully made;
your works are wonderful, I know that full well.
PSALM 139:14

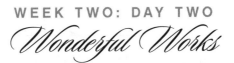

Wonderful Works

GOD AT WORK

I praise you because I am fearfully and wonderfully made;
your works are wonderful, I know that full well.
PSALM 139:14

God has always revealed himself to us through nature. I love to have my quiet time outside early in the morning. I was raised in the country and hearing the sounds of nature and smelling the fresh air does something in my spirit. I walk very early at our local high school track, and when I finish, I often drive out a country road just to watch the sun come up. When we moved to west Texas, I asked God to show me His beauty out here, and He did—and still does. I enjoy the wide-open spaces, and we have the most beautiful sunrises and sunsets. The night skies in west Texas are very dark, making the stars so visible.

Many First Place members have heard Dr. Dick Couey, a professor at Baylor University, speak at our First Place conferences. He once wrote, "If you were to count the number of stars in the sky, they would number more than the grains of sand on the Sahara Desert. The Sahara Desert is about the size of the United States—now that is a lot of stars. If you were to take the largest star and cut it into eight equal pieces, one piece would not fit between the earth and the sun."[1] What I fully know is that God's hands not only made a lot of stars, but some of them are also mighty big. God's hands are more powerful than I can fully understand. I praise Him today that I can put all of my problems in *His* hands.

Psalm 139:15 tells me that my frame is not hidden from God. These words are a comfort to me because I know that God does not make mistakes and that each of our frames is unique. You may be at your weight goal or nearing your goal and still don't have the exact shape of a model. Thank God today that He knows every inch of you and the shape you have—if you have done your part— is exactly what He planned. We may each have some flaws according to the world's opinion, but according to His Word, we are "wonderfully made." I choose to believe His Word over the world's opinion. Most of us joined First Place because we wanted to lose weight. I thought that was the only change I needed to have a perfect life. The real blessing has been His daily involvement in my personal life, and the realization of just how wonderful are His works.

Kay Smith

Take the time today to look at your surroundings and to appreciate what God's hands have made. Make note of the beauty of His creation around you. Make a list of the things in your life that you would like to commit to His hands.

Heavenly Father, I praise You today because I am fearfully and wonderfully made. Make me aware of Your daily activity in my life. I pray today to know full well just how wonderful Your works are.

I praise you because I am fearfully and wonderfully made;
your works are wonderful, I know that full well.
PSALM 139:14

Wonderful Works

NO DAYS OFF

I praise you because I am fearfully and wonderfully made;
your works are wonderful, I know that full well.
PSALM 139:14

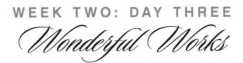

Before I came to First Place, I was a big fan of turkey and lots and lots of corn-bread dressing. Thanksgiving to me was just a food free-for-all. I would eat all day, then go home that night in misery, unbuttoning and unsnapping anything that would unbutton or unsnap. I had a very distorted view of the true meaning of Thanksgiving. In my opinion it was, "Thank You, God, for the food and a day in which to eat it. Amen." Every year I would tell myself I was going to eat anything I wanted on Thanksgiving Day and then go on a diet the day after and stick to it.

God made us fearfully and wonderfully. He knows us better than we know ourselves. I will never forget arguing with my leader the first Thanksgiving I was a member of First Place, trying to convince her that all diet programs I had ever been on allowed you to take Thanksgiving off. God knew just the kind of leadership I needed. God knew I took issues on like a bulldozer. God knew I needed to be taken down a notch or two. God knew all things about me. Most of all, God knew I was going to challenge my leader with this proposal of taking Thanksgiving off. He already had my leader in place a year before I even came to First Place, one who could stop this bulldozer in her tracks. This woman was steadfast and firm in what she believed. She looked me dead in the eye and gave me this word of wisdom that I remember to this day: "There are no days off. You don't take days off from brushing your teeth. You don't get days off to sin. There are no days off in the First Place Program. If it is to become a lifestyle, you don't take days off."

This story comes back to me each year at Thanksgiving. I took my leader's advice and stayed on the program my first Thanksgiving, and I am so thankful I did. I am thankful to God for placing strong leaders in First Place groups. I am thankful that I learned from my leader a truth that changed my life forever. If it is to become a lifestyle, there are no days off.

Beverly Henson

Day Three

Write down areas of your life in which you have been taking days off and for which you would like the Lord to help you make First Place a lifestyle.

I praise You and thank You, Father, for knowing me from the top of my head to the tip of my toes; for knowing my thoughts and having leaders in place to steer me in the right direction even before I ask the questions.

_____

_____

_____

_____

_____

_____

_____

_____

_____

_____

_____

_____

_____

_____

_____

_____

_____

_____

I praise you because I am fearfully and wonderfully made; your works are wonderful, I know that full well.
PSALM 139:14

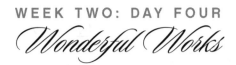

CARING FOR HIS WONDERFUL WORK

I praise you because I am fearfully and wonderfully made;
your works are wonderful, I know that full well.
PSALM 139:14

When I reached 45, I began to think that I was falling apart physically. It seemed each new week brought a new ache or pain. Within a few months it seemed I was going to the doctor every other week. Each time I had a new ailment. First it was a heel spur, then bursitis and finally I was also diagnosed with tennis elbow. On my last visit to the doctor, I suggested to the nurse that I should bring lunch the next time I came, since I saw them so regularly, and that I should make note of their birthdays as well. I felt I was now a regular member of the family at the doctor's office and, as such, needed to do my part! Getting older was beginning to really make me mad!

I shared my frustration with the doctor at having to come in to see him so often. Then he said, "Well, at least you have a different reason for coming each time. So that means I must be doing something right because whatever I prescribe works."

Boy, this young doctor was right. I was only looking at the problems and not the solutions. I had to have an attitude adjustment!

As I approach the Thanksgiving holiday, I am refocused on what wonderful works God has done on my behalf. He created me in such a wonderful way that when I feel like I am falling apart He has the prescription—the solution to my problem. Rather than being mad and frustrated with all that is wrong with my body, I have decided to do as the psalmist did and praise the Lord for His incredible handiwork! When I follow the Live-It eating plan and exercise, it is amazing how my body responds. When I take care of this body—God's wonderful work—it works the way God created it to work. God has done His wonderful, creative work, now it is up to me to take care of His wonderful work!

Nancy Taylor

Are you taking care of God's creation— your body? If not, take time to first thank Him for how wonderfully He has made you. Then list three things you can do today that will improve your life physically.

Lord, I do praise You for creating this body of mine and that it is Your wonderful work. Help me to take good care of what You have created in me.

_____

_____

_____

_____

_____

_____

_____

_____

_____

_____

_____

_____

_____

_____

_____

_____

_____

_____

I praise you because I am fearfully and wonderfully made;
your works are wonderful, I know that full well.
PSALM 139:14

Wonderful Works

FEARFULLY AND WONDERFULLY MADE

I praise you because I am fearfully and wonderfully made;
your works are wonderful, I know that full well.
PSALM 139:14

During the holidays, it is so easy to feel overworked and stressed by all the family get-togethers and extra work. Although most of us love the actual day of Thanksgiving, we don't love all the extra cleaning and cooking it entails. Even though Thanksgiving should be a time of giving thanks, we sometimes skip right over the reason we are together at this time because of all the activity.

Thanksgiving is a perfect day to give thanks to God for the family and friends He has given you. Why not invite someone who doesn't have family close by to share your meal this year? Consider starting a new family tradition of having each person present share something from the past year for which he or she is thankful.

When you feel your stress level rising this Thanksgiving, start praising and thanking God for the wonderful body He has given you. Yes, it might weigh more than you wish it did, but most likely your legs still move well enough for you to walk. Thank Him for that. Thank Him that your eyes see and that you have the ability to cook and clean. Some people without sight would give anything to be in your place. Thank God for the family you have. No family is perfect, but your family is the only one you will ever have. Thank God for the health of your family and for them being well enough to come together to celebrate the day.

Thankfulness is God's elixir for stress and feeling overworked. Thank Him for everything we have: a home, a kitchen, wonderful food to cook and eat, bodies that work well enough that we can eat and digest the food we've cooked—and the list goes on and on.

You get the point. We praise God because we are fearfully and wonderfully made. Our bodies are so wonderfully made that they begin healing when we start eating nutritious foods and exercising. Our bodies are designed to work well and are ready and waiting to heal themselves when given half a chance.

Each of us has the ability to make this Thanksgiving the best one we have ever experienced. The key is to make the entire time leading up to the actual day a time of thanks giving. On the actual day, think about why you are together with those whom you love and make it a wonderful day of giving thanks.

Carole Lewis

Think of each of your family members, starting with yourself, and write all the things for which you are thankful about each one. Being thankful will prepare you for your time together.

O Father, make this the best Thanksgiving our family has ever experienced together. Heal our hurts and make us mindful of all we have to be thankful for this year.

_____

_____

_____

_____

_____

_____

_____

_____

_____

_____

_____

_____

_____

_____

_____

_____

_____

_____

_____

I praise you because I am fearfully and wonderfully made;
your works are wonderful, I know that full well.
PSALM 139:14

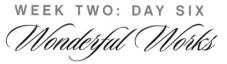

THE GENUINE PRODUCT

I praise you because I am fearfully and wonderfully made;
your works are wonderful, I know that full well.
PSALM 139:14

I remember that several years ago you would be making a fad fashion statement if you wore a Gucci watch. Gucci watches were top quality watches that had an obvious green and burgundy face, and would let others know from a distance that it was a genuine Gucci. The fine quality of these watches made the cost of these watches very high, and few people could afford them.

Before too long, we began to see what became known as knockoffs. The knockoff watch looked like a Gucci on the outside, but it wasn't even close to the quality of a genuine Gucci on the inside. Those who knew watches *knew full well* it was not a Gucci. Knockoffs could not stand the test of time like a genuine Gucci, which would seemingly last forever. A knockoff Gucci would only last a short time—until the band broke or the inner working parts stopped. You soon *knew full well* a knockoff could not equal or even come close to the quality of the genuine Gucci.

Like a fine-tuned watch, my life in Christ is genuine and recognizable as top quality. *I know full well* my body, soul and spirit are the genuine article. I was bought with a price through the precious blood of Jesus. I recognize and *know full well* all of the works of the Father in my life. I praise Him for all the victories, the breakthroughs and the strongholds that have been torn down because of His works in my life.

Through Jesus and the blood He shed for me, my life is eternal and will stand the test of time. *I know full well* that I am not a knockoff. You can tell by the look on my face to whom I belong. I am a blood-bought child of the King, royalty, an original, a genuine quality creation of my Father. I am fearfully and wonderfully made inside and out. I am the real thing.

I know full well. *I know full well.* **I KNOW FULL WELL!**

Beverly Henson

PRAYER JOURNAL: *Day Six*

List the evidences in your life for which you *know full well* that God has begun a good work in you.

I praise Your name, O Lord, for all that You have done and are doing in my life to give me more abundant life. I thank You, Father, that You have made me one of a kind. I am not a clone or a knockoff in this world. I am the genuine product, and I give You honor, praise and glory for who I am in You. I know full well that who I am today is because of You.

_____
_____
_____
_____
_____
_____
_____
_____
_____
_____
_____
_____
_____
_____
_____
_____

I praise you because I am fearfully and wonderfully made;
your works are wonderful, I know that full well.
PSALM 139:14

Wonderful Works

ORDINARY DISPENSATIONS

I praise you because I am fearfully and wonderfully made;
your works are wonderful, I know that full well.
PSALM 139:14

My copy of *Webster's Dictionary* says that Thanksgiving Day is "a public celebration to acknowledge the goodness of God, either in any remarkable deliverance from calamities or danger, or in the ordinary dispensation of his bounties."[2]

Bounty is not a word that is common to our vocabulary today, and as I looked at its meaning, "goodness" and "generosity" were two words that caught my attention. The word "bounty" brings to my mind a picture of the early Pilgrims who gave thanks to God for their bountiful harvests. It never occurred to me that God's goodness and generosity are bounties that He ordinarily dispenses to us, along with His unending mercy and love.

When my sister went home to be with the Lord after many years of suffering, some people questioned why she had to suffer for so long. Meditating on that question on the way home from her funeral, I heard on the radio a quote from Elizabeth Elliott. After losing two husbands, she said, "I do not believe in God's goodness by inference, instinct or experience. I believe in the goodness of God through faith in the Scriptures."

No matter what trials or difficulties we are currently experiencing, God's Word says that He is good and that He works all things for our good. "[His] works are wonderful, I know that full well." Through faith in the Scriptures, I know that God is good and He is worthy of our praise. "Rejoice in all the good things the LORD your God has given to you and your household" (Deuteronomy 26:11).

Think about God's goodness and generosity to you this past year. Give thanks and praise to Him this Thanksgiving season for His physical bounties and also for the goodness and generosity that are ordinary dispensations from God to His children.

Pat Lewis

Day Seven

Chronicle in your journal the things *you know full well* about God: His faithfulness, His love, His kindness, His goodness and how He has revealed these character traits in your life.

Father, I thank You today for Your wonderful bounties of goodness and generosity that You dispense to me on a daily basis, along with my physical needs. Thank You that my circumstances do not determine Your goodness. You are always good and worthy to be praised. There is no time when You are not good. Thank You for Your Word that is always true and faithful.

_____
_____
_____
_____
_____
_____
_____
_____
_____
_____
_____
_____
_____
_____
_____
_____
_____
_____

I praise you because I am fearfully and wonderfully made;
your works are wonderful, I know that full well.
Psalm 139:14

Birth of a Savior

MANGER TO A CROSS

For to us a child is born, to us a son is given,
and the government will be on his shoulders.
And he will be called Wonderful Counselor,
Mighty God, Everlasting Father, Prince of Peace.
ISAIAH 9:6

The church was packed for the first performance of our Christmas pageant "His Kingdom." This was my first experience being in such a huge production. We had worked very hard for the past few months, and our family lives had revolved around the practice schedule. It was truly a blessing just to show up for practice and be a part of all the music and drama, the beautiful Victorian dresses, makeup artists, and wardrobe persons. What excitement! I began to feel as if I were part of a Broadway production.

We were about midway through the performance that first evening when an awesome thing happened. This particular scene highlighted a cast member carrying a manger from the back of the sanctuary up the aisle to the front of the church. Dramatic music filled the sanctuary as he entered with the manger. As he made the turn up the aisle, he lifted the manger high over his head and a bright light shone on it, which caused a huge silhouette on the wall. Amazingly, it was not the silhouette of a manger but of a *cross*! Only a few in the cast could see this, but as he turned into the aisle to move to the front, the silhouette only enlarged and changed the angle of the cross. Now, it caught the attention of everyone. It was such an "oh, wow!" moment. The light was shining on a manger, but there was a 20-foot cross on the wall!

I immediately realized that God was reminding us to focus on the cross. The nativity story is so heartwarming and miraculous, but it's the cross that changed my life. It's the cross that gave me salvation, secured my eternity and gives me strength for today. It was an awesome moment. I never see a manger that I am not reminded of that pageant and the unexpected cross. When I see a baby in the manger, I thank God for a baby that grew up and died on the cross to cover my sins. I never make the mistake of leaving Jesus in a manger. His death makes me acceptable in God's presence. His blood covers my sins. What a tremendous gift that we are given the opportunity to accept, which I did at a young age. It was not until I became a mother that I fully realized the depth of that love. God's love is often beyond my understanding, but never beyond my reach.

Kay Smith

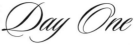

Describe your salvation experience. Your testimony is power against Satan's attacks. If you have never accepted Jesus Christ as your Savior, pray to do so right now. Accept the greatest gift ever given. Use Romans 3:23; 5:8; 6:23; 10:9-10 to direct you.

Thank You, God, for the precious gift of Jesus Christ. Teach me how to daily use the power that I am promised by His sacrifice on the cross.

_____

_____

_____

_____

_____

_____

_____

_____

_____

_____

_____

_____

_____

_____

_____

_____

_____

_____

For to us a child is born, to us a son is given,
and the government will be on his shoulders.
And he will be called Wonderful Counselor,
Mighty God, Everlasting Father, Prince of Peace.
Isaiah 9:6

Birth of a Savior

HOW MANY NAMES DO YOU HAVE?

For to us a child is born, to us a son is given,
and the government will be on his shoulders.
And he will be called Wonderful Counselor,
Mighty God, Everlasting Father, Prince of Peace.
ISAIAH 9:6

Christmas time is a busy time with shopping, baking, parties and decorating. However, life as a mom, wife, daughter and friend is always busy! It seems I am continually taking on a new title. This year, along with being Mom to my 17-year-old daughter, I took on the title of "Team Mom." I now have the responsibility of not only encouraging my daughter but also of encouraging all 12 team members! I must see that each team member has a snack and a note of encouragement before the game, and that the concession stand is manned for the games. This—on top of a full-time job and a family to care for—has caused a few stressful moments. I suppose that as a woman, I was born for all these titles that have been given to me.

When Jesus was born, He was given many names and many tasks. He was born with the names Wonderful Counselor, Mighty God, Eternal Father and Prince of Peace. Can you imagine the tasks that those names imply? The names of Mom, daughter, Nancy, wife bring about overwhelming responsibilities for me, yet Jesus is never overwhelmed with the tasks of His divine nature. During these stressful days, we can cast our anxieties on Him and He will carry our load *plus* His. That is amazing and comforting!

Team Mom was becoming a burden, but when I prayed and asked the Mighty God for help, He provided several other moms who volunteered to come alongside me and share the various tasks set before us. The burden has lifted and He has given me rest (see Matthew 11:28-30). When I call on His name, He provides all I need to live out the many names that I have been given. He is wonderful!

Nancy Taylor

List all the titles you have been given and responsibilities that you are called to do. Pray for each name and responsibility, specifically asking God to provide through His powerful names.

I praise You, my Wonderful Counselor, Mighty God, Eternal Father and Prince of Peace. Thank You for being faithful to Your names and providing all I need to live out the tasks that You call me to do.

_____

_____

_____

_____

_____

_____

_____

_____

_____

_____

_____

_____

_____

_____

_____

_____

_____

_____

_____

For to us a child is born, to us a son is given,
and the government will be on his shoulders.
And he will be called Wonderful Counselor,
Mighty God, Everlasting Father, Prince of Peace.
ISAIAH 9:6

Birth of a Savior

THE WHOLE PICTURE

For to us a child is born, to us a son is given,
and the government will be on his shoulders.
And he will be called Wonderful Counselor,
Mighty God, Everlasting Father, Prince of Peace.
ISAIAH 9:6

I don't know about you, but when I read this verse, the first thing I did was sigh a big sigh of exhaustion just thinking about the responsibility that is upon Jesus: "The government will be on his shoulders." What a horrible burden for Him to carry. Where's the joy that this Scripture is really talking about? Shouldn't there be a lot more than a feeling of burden that accompanies a baby being born: the security of having an everlasting Father, the relief of knowing we have a wonderful Counselor, the safety of a mighty God, the rest that is afforded to us because the Prince of peace lives within us? Of course, I just have to look on a bit further to see the bigger picture.

Do you sometimes get stuck in your nearsighted view of the situation instead of seeing the whole picture? Do you go through life like this or, more specifically, at the holidays? The holidays sure can be tough on people and may be especially tough for you this year. Often, sadness can be caused by comparison: Does everyone have it better than me? They are prettier, wealthier and much happier. They have better cars, marriages and families. They have more Christmas cards, more gifts under the tree, more parties to attend, etc. Get my drift?

Our thinking is what gets us into trouble. One little peek at the couple next door and the picture painted is a perfect, happy life. The Lord is teaching me to look up instead of looking around. When I am looking up, there is nothing to distract me from focusing on MY Prince of Peace, MY Wonderful Counselor, MY Mighty God or MY Everlasting Father. The only person for whom I have to answer to God is me! I am learning that the sooner I quit looking at my little view of the picture and start trusting the Artist who knows far better the picture being painted, the more peaceful I will be.

What is the picture you are seeing this holiday?

Stephanie Cheves

What have you been looking at this holiday? List everything that has taken up your time and attention. Cross out all those things that are beyond God's control. Then write out a prayer of thanksgiving for all that Jesus offers through His very name.

Lord, forgive me for being short-sighted, not seeing the whole picture. Thank You that You are able to carry the burden of the whole world along with my own personal anxieties.

_____

_____

_____

_____

_____

_____

_____

_____

_____

_____

_____

_____

_____

_____

_____

_____

_____

For to us a child is born, to us a son is given,
and the government will be on his shoulders.
And he will be called Wonderful Counselor,
Mighty God, Everlasting Father, Prince of Peace.
ISAIAH 9:6

Birth of a Savior

WHAT'S IN A NAME?

For to us a child is born, to us a son is given,
and the government will be on his shoulders.
And he will be called Wonderful Counselor,
Mighty God, Everlasting Father, Prince of Peace.
ISAIAH 9:6

There is nothing more miraculous than childbirth. What mother can ever forget the moment her child was born and placed in her arms? After much pain and suffering, a child is born; a son or daughter is given to you. The joy, peace and love that overflows your heart is indescribable. Looking at your beautiful newborn baby, you think, *What will be his name, what shall we call him?* With today's modern technology, most parents know soon after conception if their child is a boy or girl. Many decide what the name will be and begin to call their child by that name long before birth.

In ancient times, names were given to indicate function, character and destiny. When my children were born, it was common to give popular names without much thought to their meaning. Today the trend has returned to biblical names. A recent newspaper article said that Joshua and Jacob are among the most popular biblical names for boys. Whatever name we are given, it is unique to our person, distinguishing us from others. However, even though our child has a given name, we sometimes call him or her by an affectionate name, or perhaps a nickname.

This week's Scripture says that Jesus was called by many names: Wonderful Counselor, Mighty God, Everlasting Father, Prince of Peace. These names not only describe who He was but also His function, His character and His destiny. The Bible also says that He has a name that is above every name (see Philippians 2:9).

One morning as I was reading 1 John 3, I was awestruck by the first verse: "How great is the love the Father has lavished on us, that we should be called children of God! And that is what we are!" The name given to us by our parents is our earthly name, but God calls us by His name, one that defines our function, character and destiny as His children.

"Yet to all who received him, to those who believed in his name, he gave the right to become children of God" (John 1:12). What an awesome privilege and responsibility to be called His children.

Pat Lewis

Ask God to search your heart today to see if there is anything associated with your earthly name that does not bring honor and glory to the name of Jesus. Receive God's forgiveness and thank Him for His mercy.

O Lord, our Lord, how excellent is Your name in all the earth. What an honor to be called by Your name. Help me to live a life that will always honor and glorify Your name on this earth.

_____

_____

_____

_____

_____

_____

_____

_____

_____

_____

_____

_____

_____

_____

_____

_____

For to us a child is born, to us a son is given,
and the government will be on his shoulders.
And he will be called Wonderful Counselor,
Mighty God, Everlasting Father, Prince of Peace.
ISAIAH 9:6

Birth of a Savior

PRECIOUS MOMENTS

For to us a child is born, to us a son is given,
and the government will be on his shoulders.
And he will be called Wonderful Counselor,
Mighty God, Everlasting Father, Prince of Peace.
ISAIAH 9:6

When each of our children were born, it was a time of rejoicing. All three were born healthy, with 10 fingers and 10 toes and all their facial parts in the right place. Johnny and I and, of course, both sets of grandparents, along with aunts and uncles, used descriptive words such as "beautiful," "perfect," "adorable," "precious" and "sweet" to describe our babies.

Every time a wanted child is born into the world it is a time of rejoicing, but when Jesus the Christ was born, it was a time like no other. Let's look at the words used to describe this blessed baby:

- **Wonderful**—Nothing this wonderful had happened in the entire world since God created it. Wonderful was a descriptive name given to Jesus because He alone was to be the conduit whereby our lives now had the potential to be wonderful because of Him.
- **Counselor**—All the professional counselors in the world could never match the counseling that Jesus Christ gives to those who ask Him.
- **Mighty God**—Mighty God came to Earth in the form of a little baby so that we might see flesh and blood deity. The Bible is our guidebook about our mighty God becoming man.
- **Everlasting Father**—This baby—by living among us, dying on the cross for our sins and arising from the grave—insured that He was now our way of living eternally. We can receive our everlasting Father just by accepting Jesus into our life.
- **Prince of Peace**—Our God is a God of peace (see 1 Thessalonians 5:23), and His Son, Jesus, is the Prince of Peace. Knowing this Prince of Peace is where true peace is found.

Make this Christmas the best one ever by recognizing the difference this blessed Baby can make in your own life, if you will only ask Him in. Jesus desires to be Wonderful in your life. He wants to be your Counselor. He desires to show Himself mighty in your life. He wants to be your Father forever. His desire is to come in and bring peace amidst the chaos.

Make room for Christ in your Christmas this year and you will never be the same!

Carole Lewis

Begin by writing each of these descriptive names given to Jesus when He was born. After each name write your thankfulness, needs and desires for this particular name to become reality in your life.

Dear Jesus, I want to love You so much that all of Your descriptive names become a part of who I am. Draw close to me as I draw close to You.

_____

_____

_____

_____

_____

_____

_____

_____

_____

_____

_____

_____

_____

_____

_____

_____

_____

_____

_____

_____

For to us a child is born, to us a son is given,
and the government will be on his shoulders.
And he will be called Wonderful Counselor,
Mighty God, Everlasting Father, Prince of Peace.
ISAIAH 9:6

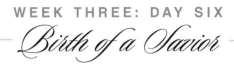
Birth of a Savior

THE BREAD OF LIFE

For to us a child is born, to us a son is given,
and the government will be on his shoulders.
And he will be called Wonderful Counselor,
Mighty God, Everlasting Father, Prince of Peace.
ISAIAH 9:6

Christmas is a twinkling time of year for me. I love the decorations and the glitter. The spirit of giving is so prevailing during the Christmas season that even those who do not consider themselves religious unknowingly get caught up in the precious spirit of the season. I love the fact that we still celebrate Christmas as the door God opened to introduce His Son to this world "that [we] might have life and that [we] might have it more abundantly" (John 10:10, *KJV*).

As I was studying to become certified as a personal trainer, my studies took me into an area of sports nutrition. An area I was particularly interested in was carbohydrates. Carbohydrates are the fuel for our body. We have to have them to effectively go about our daily task. In First Place we know carbohydrates as our bread exchanges.

It happened to be at Christmastime that I was reading this information. I rested my book in my lap and looked at the nativity set on my coffee table. I saw the baby Jesus lying in the manger. And what was the manger? It was a feed trough with the Bread of Life lying in it. God had given the world a Savior, who is Christ the Lord. Jesus didn't refer to himself as the Meat of Life. He didn't refer to himself as the Vegetable of Life. He referred to himself as the Bread of Life because Jesus is the fuel my spiritual body needs each day to be effective for Him as I go about my daily tasks. The manger was the humble serving platter on which God presented the Bread of Life to the world.

As you are filling out your Commitment Record this Christmas season, take a moment when you come to the line for the bread exchange and think about the Bread exchange God gave you when He gave you His Son, Jesus. Jesus is the fuel that gets you through each day. He truly is your Bread of Life.

Beverly Henson

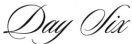
Write down the tasks you have ahead of you today for which you could use a little extra fuel. Write a prayer asking God to give you the fuel you need to sustain you today as you tackle these tasks.

Thank You, Father, for giving me the Bread of Life for fuel to make it through this day.

_____

_____

_____

_____

_____

_____

_____

_____

_____

_____

_____

_____

_____

_____

_____

_____

_____

_____

_____

For to us a child is born, to us a son is given,
and the government will be on his shoulders.
And he will be called Wonderful Counselor,
Mighty God, Everlasting Father, Prince of Peace.
Isaiah 9:6

Birth of a Savior

GOD'S GIFTS

For to us a child is born, to us a son is given,
and the government will be on his shoulders.
And he will be called Wonderful Counselor,
Mighty God, Everlasting Father, Prince of Peace.
ISAIAH 9:6

I envision four large, beautifully wrapped Christmas presents sitting under our lovely, glistening Christmas tree. The first gift represents Jesus as my Wonderful Counselor. When I need advice, I go to Him and He answers all my questions and gives me instructions for each day. I once told God that I didn't feel like I was anyone's favorite person. He led me to John 3:16 and as I read those words I heard a small voice say, "You are my favorite. Isn't that enough?" Yes, it was.

The second gift represents Mighty God, more powerful than any of my enemies and promising victory in all battles if I stay in His will. I have a history with God. He has done things in my life that are superhuman. I realize now that David was a giant slayer before he went into that valley to fight Goliath because he knew the battle belonged to the Lord. He was just there to swing a slingshot.

The third reminds me that God is my Everlasting Father. It was easy for me to accept God as Father because I could relate Him to my earthly father. My dad was a quiet, strong man with tender hands that combed my long curly hair without ever pulling. He was always on my side, even if I had been wrong. He gave me a strong desire to do well because of his love and trust in me. But one Sunday afternoon 20-plus years ago, I got a very unexpected call. My dad had carried out the trash, come back in the door, gone into the bathroom and died of a massive heart attack. He was gone: I could no longer tell him the stories of our daily lives; I couldn't kiss his cheek and see his slight smile. He was no longer quietly sitting at the end of the kitchen table, where he would be in the center of activity. I wanted to scream that this was so unfair! And I did. My dad, as good as he was, was only an example of God's love for me. He was gone now. I now understand the huge blessing of an Everlasting Father never out of my presence—always ready to hear my stories and give me advice.

The fourth present represents the peace God gives me when I rest in Him. But look! There is a fifth present—not as large or as pretty. This gift represents what I have to give God—my life—giving Him permission to be the ruler. It is only when I allow the government of my life to be on His shoulders that I can enjoy this huge gift of peace, resting because of His promises and His directions, His power and His everlasting presence in my life.

Kay Smith

List the ways that you know these gifts have also been given to you. You may have areas in your life that you have not yet given to God. Ask Him to identify those areas and give them to Him today.

Thank You, God, for these four gifts in my life. Help me to open and enjoy them especially today. Thank You for accepting the gift of my life. Help me to fully give my life to You. Give me Your instruction, Your power, the knowledge of Your presence and Your peace today.

For to us a child is born, to us a son is given,
and the government will be on his shoulders.
And he will be called Wonderful Counselor,
Mighty God, Everlasting Father, Prince of Peace.
ISAIAH 9:6

Gift of Love

BEING LOVED

*This is love: not that we loved God, but that he loved us
and sent his Son as an atoning sacrifice for our sins.*
1 JOHN 4:10

When my son was 15 years old, he struggled with his self-image and sense of worth. He would spend hours in his room all alone with his thoughts. He spiraled down into depression with thoughts of suicide. My husband and I had raised our children in what we thought was a loving Christian home. We would praise our son with words of affirmation, but they would fall on deaf ears. He would not accept our love or our encouraging words. He was angry with everyone and spoke only words of hatred and disgust to his family. We were at our wits' end until we realized the need to pray Scripture for our son. I began to pray Ephesians 3:16-19 for him in this way: "Lord, I pray that You would grant him according to the riches of Your glory to be strengthened with power through Your Spirit in his inner man, so that Christ would dwell in his heart and that he would be rooted and grounded in love and that he would be able to comprehend the breadth and length and height and depth of Your love." Over the next month, I diligently prayed this truth into the life of my son.

God's love miraculously changed my son's heart and life. He finally accepted God's love and began to grasp its expanse. He began to write songs of God's mercy, grace and love and shared them as he led worship at his school each week. A total transformation took place. Because he had accepted God's love, he was then, in turn, able to love others. Just loving others or even loving God is not love at all. According to 1 John 4:10, love can only flow from us after we have accepted the unconditional and sacrificial love that the Father has for us.

Christmas is a time for loving others, giving to others and celebrating the love of the Father represented in the birth of Jesus. Take time each day to fill up with the truth of God's Word that He loves you. Bask in His love and enjoy how truly vast it is. Then you will be filled up and ready to give out to others this God-given love.

Nancy Taylor

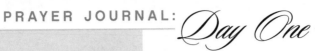

Make a list of all the ways God has shown His love for you. Spend time meditating on the truth of 1 John 4:10, writing out ways you can show His love to others this Christmas.

Thank You, Lord, for loving me so much that You sent Jesus as a sacrifice for my sins. How great a love You have for me that You would give Your one and only Son that I might live eternally with You, forever experiencing Your love.

_____

_____

_____

_____

_____

_____

_____

_____

_____

_____

_____

_____

_____

_____

_____

_____

_____

This is love: not that we loved God, but that he loved us and sent his Son as an atoning sacrifice for our sins.
1 John 4:10

Gift of Love

HE PAID THE PRICE

This is love: not that we loved God, but that he loved us
and sent his Son as an atoning sacrifice for our sins.
1 JOHN 4:10

To atone for something is to pay for mistakes made or sins committed. When you break a law, you are expected to pay a penalty for the crime. When you make a mistake, there is a cost involved in correcting the mistake. I recently browsed through a gift shop that had a sign posted at the cash register that said, "You break it, you buy it!" I grew up with parents who taught me that if I made a mess, I was to clean it up. I found this also to be true with my weight management. I would go on an emotional eating binge and then a month later find myself 10 pounds heavier. I was a yo-yo dieter for years and would often join a well-known weight loss center to lose weight. They would have us say each week before leaving the meeting, "If it is to be, then it is up to me!" In other words, it was my responsibility to clean up my mess and to pay for my lack of self-control. I found myself in a never-ending cycle of guilt, self-condemnation and frustration.

Are you ready for the rest of the story? I found hope and healing in the knowledge that God had paid for my sins and my mistakes by sending His one and only Son, Jesus Christ, as an atoning sacrifice once and for all! He paid the price for my mistakes, for my sin, even though He was sinless! It was as if I had broken the figurine in the gift shop, and the owner not only paid for the broken figurine but also gave me a brand new one in its place! It was my fault, yet he took responsibility for it. I had overeaten and not taken care of my body, yet when I cried to the Lord and asked for His strength, He provided all that I needed to overcome the cycle of sin in my life. This week's Scripture verse gives me motivation in my pursuit of physical wellness. Knowing that Jesus paid the price for my past, present and future sins motivates me to honor Him with my body (see 1 Corinthians 6:19-20).

He paid the price, and now it is my joy to honor Him by taking care of this body that He redeemed with His precious Son. During this Christmas season, may each gift given and each gift received remind you of the costly and precious gift of life that God has given you and may you give Him in return a life that honors Him.

Nancy Taylor

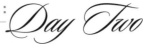

Is there something that you are trying to accomplish in your own strength? Describe the situation. Are you trying to correct a mistake that you have made following your own plan? Explain. Accept God's payment for your mistakes and sins and ask the Lord to give you His wisdom and strength to overcome any hindrance in your life. Write your prayer in this journal.

Lord, I can never repay You for redeeming me from a life of guilt, self-condemnation and frustration. Thank You for Your mercy and Your grace. May my life bring honor to You.

_____

_____

_____

_____

_____

_____

_____

_____

_____

_____

_____

_____

_____

_____

_____

_____

This is love: not that we loved God, but that he loved us and sent his Son as an atoning sacrifice for our sins.
1 John 4:10

Gift of Love

LOVE IS A CHOICE

*This is love: not that we loved God, but that he loved us
and sent his Son as an atoning sacrifice for our sins.*
1 JOHN 4:10

I hear people grumble as the Christmas decorations seem to appear in the stores earlier and earlier each year, but I am not one of those people. I think we should leave the decorations out all year. I love to walk in a store and see all the beautiful decorations with Christmas music filling the air. I just sense more love in the air at this time of the year. Maybe it is because we focus on others by giving gifts, planning parties and communicating with friends and family.

Shopping may be depressing for some. Time is short and money even shorter. Our verse this week suggests a Christmas gift that surpasses all others. Christmas may bring us together with family and friends, which might include some people whom we find difficult to love. On occasion, I have mentioned to God that I would love these people, but they really should acknowledge how much they have hurt me in the past. In some cases, it is more the way they behave now that causes the problem. I believe that if God would just set them straight, I could really love them. Then I see this verse, and I realize that God has set the standard. My job is just to love them, but it will only happen in His power.

God's Word is teaching me that love is more than a good feeling. His Word motivates me to respond in ways that emulate His goodness. Love sometimes demands that I act in very practical and even uncomfortable ways.

Love is not an option; we are commanded to love one another (see 1 John 3:11). Love is demonstrative (see 1 John 3:16). Love is an act of the will (see 1 John 3:18). I have learned that to follow God's instruction, I often have to act a certain way, even though I do not feel like it. Zig Ziglar once said, "It is easier to act your way into a new way of feeling than it is to feel your way into a new way of acting." Love is responsive (see 1 John 4:19). We are able to love because we have been loved and are loved by God. I think if we use the Cross as the backdrop to any circumstance we are facing, we can give love.

The gift of love we give to others provides the assurance that we have moved away from the way of darkness and death and toward the way of light and life (see 1 John 2:8-11). It seems to me that if I choose to give the gift of love to someone this holiday, it will bless me—because I have been obedient—and it will glorify God. I cannot come up with a better gift idea, and the price has already been paid.

Kay Smith

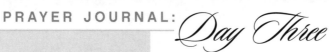
List the people in your life whom you find hard to love. Tell God what it is that makes it hard to love them. List specific ways that you could show love to each person you listed.

Heavenly Father, thank You for the gift of love You have given me. Please reveal to me the people in my life who need my gift of love. I need Your wisdom and Your strength to be obedient to Your command for me to love others this holiday season.

_____

_____

_____

_____

_____

_____

_____

_____

_____

_____

_____

_____

_____

_____

_____

_____

This is love: not that we loved God, but that he loved us and sent his Son as an atoning sacrifice for our sins.
1 JOHN 4:10

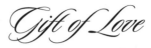

NO QUESTIONS ASKED

This is love: not that we loved God, but that he loved us
and sent his Son as an atoning sacrifice for our sins.
1 JOHN 4:10

What is your definition of love? What's your perception of love? How do you express love, and how is it expressed to you? You might have noticed that 1 John 4:10 does not ask any of these questions. It states God's definition of love, gives the truest view of love and explains how our heavenly Father has demonstrated His love toward us. No questions asked.

He knew where we would be today. He knows that sometimes we may struggle with accepting being loved, but He is not asking us any questions about it. He is telling us what love is and what He is offering us because of His love. Isn't that just like God to dot the *I*s and cross the *T*s? His love for us is not dependent on our understanding of it, our attitude toward him or our definition of it. Love is JESUS CHRIST.

Can you think of anything more amazing than the King of kings loving you unconditionally? So often, we are manipulated by this world, and unfortunately love is one of the most twisted offerings out there. "If you love me, you will do this" is so often the message. It's as though love is dangled before us like a carrot, and it's only given when we meet the other person's requirements—unlike Jesus, worldly love is not a gift. God never dangles Christ before us as a carrot. He gives His love freely, and the only condition is that we accept His gift of Jesus Christ.

Jesus is truly a gift to us so that we can come to our heavenly Father.

Will you accept His love this Christmas—no questions asked?

Stephanie Cheves

Have you been unwilling to love others unconditionally? Have you put requirements on your love? Confess this to the Father and make a list of ways you can demonstrate God's love to others.

Lord, thank You for Your gift of love in the form of Jesus Christ. I accept His love for me today with no questions asked.

_____

_____

_____

_____

_____

_____

_____

_____

_____

_____

_____

_____

_____

_____

_____

_____

_____

_____

_____

This is love: not that we loved God, but that he loved us and sent his Son as an atoning sacrifice for our sins.
1 JOHN 4:10

Gift of Love

EXTRAVAGANT LOVE

This is love: not that we loved God, but that he loved us
and sent his Son as an atoning sacrifice for our sins.
1 JOHN 4:10

Christmas is my favorite time of year. I love all the twinkling lights, the joyful music about the birth of our Savior, the atmosphere of love and giving of gifts, home and family, the midnight Christmas Eve service at the church, and all the traditions that we have come to know and associate with the Christmas season.

One of my favorite childhood memories is of the Christmas Eve program at our church. There was a large Christmas tree that all the church members helped decorate, little shepherd children, angels with cardboard wings, Mary and Joseph and baby Jesus, plus all the traditional Christmas carols. In the audience were those who had traveled home to spend Christmas with their families. It was an exciting and memorable event for me as a child, especially during a time when my parents were unable to lavish us children with many gifts.

A few years ago I heard of a group of people who determined that celebrating Christmas, giving gifts and decorating a Christmas tree was associated with paganism and that Christians should not participate in this celebration. One day during that Christmas season, I was driving to a friend's home and was talking to the Lord about Christmas and how much I enjoyed the time of year. I asked Him what He thought about Christmas. He spoke to my spirit and said, "Christmas is a time of love," adding that He loved the world so much that He gave His one and only Son that whoever would believe in Him shall not perish but have eternal life (see John 3:16).

God loved and He gave. That's why we can joyfully celebrate the Christmas season by loving others and giving gifts as an outflow of that love. Giving is a natural outflow from a heart that deeply loves. It is not important if the date of Jesus' birth is exact, but it does matter to God that we love and sacrifice our lives for one another, not only at Christmas but also all year long.

Let the light of the love of Jesus twinkle in your heart and shine in your countenance as you celebrate the Christmas season. Observe how Christ loved us. His love is not cautious but extravagant. He didn't love in order to get something from us but to give everything of Himself to us. Love like that!

Pat Lewis

PRAYER JOURNAL: *Day Five*

Write a love letter to God. Ask God to fill your heart with love for any difficult-to-love person in your life.

Thank You, Father, that You loved us so much that You gave Your only Son as a sacrifice so that we could live with You forever. Thank You that Your love is in our hearts so that we can love our neighbor as ourselves.

This is love: not that we loved God, but that he loved us and sent his Son as an atoning sacrifice for our sins.
1 JOHN 4:10

Gift of Love

A JUST-BECAUSE LOVE

This is love: not that we loved God, but that he loved us
and sent his Son as an atoning sacrifice for our sins.
1 JOHN 4:10

The greatest gift I can give myself is to come to the realization and the revelation of just how much God loves me! He loves me just because. It is not conditional on the fact that I lost 147 pounds or that I lost 14 pounds. He loves me just because. I had not lost one pound when I began to realize exactly how much He really does love me.

The revelation of His love came to me at the First Place Conference in New Orleans. I was at the end of my rope and had exhausted all hope. Weighing nearly 300 pounds, I thought I was destined to grow old and always be overweight. Before the conference I prayed, *Father, let me find the answers I have been desperately seeking.*

The first thing I remember when I went into the sanctuary was that the pews were so close together. I wondered if I would be able to fit. I had to stand on my toes so that my stomach would clear the opening. I hoped I would not have to leave my seat often because I was exhausted from just sitting down. The conference was great, and I enjoyed it very much. After the morning session I found myself talking to Dr. Dick Couey. The prayer I had prayed was about to be answered. He gave me some tips to raise my metabolism. The tips all involved exercise, and I refused to hear what he had told me. He then looked straight in my eyes and said something I had never heard, "You can stay just like you are, and God is going to love you anyway, or you can go home and make the changes."

God was going to love me whether I weighed 300 pounds or 100 pounds! The only thing that ever mattered to me was weight loss and pounds. I was free because weight loss and pounds do not affect how much God loves me. He loves me just because! I felt as if God had breathed new life into me. I let go of weight and pounds and took hold of the fact that He loves me.

This Christmas season let God breathe that fresh breath on you and embrace the precious love He gave to the world through the gift of His Son, Jesus.

Beverly Henson

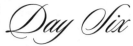
Read the prayer I asked before the conference; then write it down and list the areas of your life in which you are seeking answers.

Father, breathe a fresh breath of love on me today.

_____

_____

_____

_____

_____

_____

_____

_____

_____

_____

_____

_____

_____

_____

_____

_____

_____

_____

_____

_____

_____

This is love: not that we loved God, but that he loved us and sent his Son as an atoning sacrifice for our sins.
1 JOHN 4:10

Gift of Love

THE BEST CHRISTMAS GIFT

This is love: not that we loved God, but that he loved us
and sent his Son as an atoning sacrifice for our sins.
1 JOHN 4:10

The movie *The Passion of the Christ* was first released just before Easter 2004. Our church reserved an entire theater before the movie's debut so that our church staff could see the film first and be able to answer questions we might be asked after others viewed the film. Because of all the reports we had read about the movie, Johnny and I arrived feeling just a little anxious and unsure of what might be in store. We certainly didn't buy anything to munch on during the film because it seemed totally out of place for this particular film.

After the film was over, no one in the entire audience was able to move—let alone stand and leave the theater. Our pastor walked to the front and led us in prayer. After his prayer, we all stood hesitantly and made our way out. No one uttered a word as we departed, but most of the women ended up in the restroom together and what a mess we all were. Our makeup was streaked and our eyes were swollen from crying during the depiction of the suffering of the Lord Jesus.

I'm sure that each of us love our children enough to die for them if they were in danger. We would jump into a raging river or run into a burning house to save the life of our own child. However, there is probably not a single person reading this today who would love another person enough to sacrifice his or her own child to save that person's life.

Jesus' sole purpose of coming to this earth and being born as a baby was to become the atoning sacrifice for your sin and mine. Mull over the kind of love displayed by the God of heaven when He sent Jesus to Earth. Jesus was willing to leave the splendor of heaven so that each of us could one day spend eternity there with Him.

This Christmas look at the birth of that tiny baby in a new way. God became flesh and dwelt among us so that we might truly know Him. The best part of knowing Jesus is the power He gives us to endure the hardships and suffering of our fallen world. Better than that is being able to live a victorious life in spite of our sins and shortcomings. Now that's some kind of love!

Carole Lewis

Spend some time reflecting on the kind of love God had for you that would cause Him to allow His one and only Son, Jesus, to come to Earth to die for your sins. Ask God to make you very aware of His presence this Christmas season.

Dear God, I want to thank You for being willing to send Your one and only Son, Jesus, into this world. Thank You, Jesus, for being willing to come and die for my sins. Thank You that Your death has the power to give me victory over the sin in my life.

_____

_____

_____

_____

_____

_____

_____

_____

_____

_____

_____

_____

_____

_____

_____

_____

_____

This is love: not that we loved God, but that he loved us and sent his Son as an atoning sacrifice for our sins.
1 JOHN 4:10

Spring Forward

ALL OR NOTHING

Forget the former things; do not dwell on the past.
See, I am doing a new thing! Now it springs up; do you not perceive it?
I am making a way in the desert and streams in the wasteland.
ISAIAH 43:18-19

I am the queen of all or nothing! I might decide on Monday that I am going to start doing all nine commitments. I mean it. This Monday, I will do it. Well, you probably know where this is going; by Tuesday, yep, I've messed up so I will just have to wait until next Monday to start again. So that means another whole week of dwelling on my slipup and from here I go to the next thing I didn't do that I thought would—and so it begins. I begin remembering the past, and usually it's not the good things. Now what happens? I get down and decide I am the worst person ever. I can't keep one commitment let alone *nine*! Remember that one time I said something the wrong way? Well, I should never speak again—I am the worst! And what about that time when . . .

Do you do this? Do you beat yourself up because of the past? Well, *stop* it! So we make a mistake here and there. Is it the end of the world? Of course not. If it were the end of the world, I am pretty sure you had nothing to do with it, and it's not a mistake.

The new year is the time we declare our plans for the upcoming year. It is not to keep looking back and focusing on the past. If I am constantly looking back, won't it be rather difficult to move forward? Think of what happens when you walk while looking backward; you zigzag, run into things and are hesitant to move. This is no way to follow Christ. When we are truly following Christ, we won't have time to look back.

Remember the saying, "You are not responsible for what comes into your mind, but you are responsible for how long it stays"? This new year let's keep our eyes on Christ *leading* us through the desert and streams, not on what's in the past.

Stephanie Cheves

List some short-term goals for this week. Write a prayer asking God to supply all that you need to meet these goals.

Lord, keep me focused on today and what it is You would have me do. Lord, forgive me for looking back. I ask now that You would continue to show me the path to follow each day.

_____
_____
_____
_____
_____
_____
_____
_____
_____
_____
_____
_____
_____
_____
_____
_____
_____
_____
_____

Forget the former things; do not dwell on the past.
See, I am doing a new thing! Now it springs up; do you not perceive it?
I am making a way in the desert and streams in the wasteland.
ISAIAH 43:18-19

Spring Forward

NEW THINGS

Forget the former things; do not dwell on the past.
See, I am doing a new thing! Now it springs up; do you not perceive it?
I am making a way in the desert and streams in the wasteland.
ISAIAH 43:18-19

Don't you just love new things? They are fresh, clean and without any spots and stains. About a year after my husband went home to heaven, I sold our home and moved to a new, smaller home in a new neighborhood. I put new paint on the walls, new carpet and tile on the floors, hung new doors, and even bought some new furniture. I left behind the former things and became excited about new things. I prayed that God would show me a new plan for my life and fill my life with new things.

My late husband told me of a time he was counseling with a married couple and discovered they were still fighting over an incident that happened on their wedding day 25 years before. How many of us spend valuable days, hours and minutes dwelling on former things: wounds received through harsh words, unkind deeds, wrongs committed against us. I've heard it said that "before you can move on, you must face the disappointments of the past. To stay stuck in the past will rob you of the blessings of the future."

God has much to say about old and new things. Ephesians 4:22-24 says, "You were taught, with regard to your former way of life, to put off your old self, which is being corrupted by its deceitful desires; to be made new in the attitude of your minds; and to put on the new self, created to be like God in true righteousness and holiness." Isaiah 65:17 says, "Behold, I will create new heavens and a new earth. The former things will not be remembered, nor will they come to mind."

Carole Lewis tells of her mom who would wake up every morning after her dad died and say, "God, what wonderful new things do you have for me today?" What a great example of not dwelling on the past but on looking forward to new and exciting things God wants to do in our lives.

God gives us each a new day and a new year filled with exciting new things for us to enjoy. New things will spring up in our paths if we are willing to forget the things that caused pain this past year and focus on the new things God has planned for us.

Pat Lewis

List the things in your past that you are still dwelling on or remembering with hurt or anger, and give them up to God today as an offering of forgiveness toward those who may have caused the pain. Ask God to show you new and exciting things He wants to do in your life.

Thank You, Lord, for new things in our lives. Help us to not dwell on the past but to look forward to the wonderful things You have planned for each new day.

_____

_____

_____

_____

_____

_____

_____

_____

_____

_____

_____

_____

_____

_____

_____

_____

_____

Forget the former things; do not dwell on the past.
See, I am doing a new thing! Now it springs up; do you not perceive it?
I am making a way in the desert and streams in the wasteland.
ISAIAH 43:18-19

Spring Forward

PHEW! A NEW THING!

Forget the former things; do not dwell on the past.
See, I am doing a new thing! Now it springs up; do you not perceive it?
I am making a way in the desert and streams in the wasteland.
ISAIAH 43:18-19

Have you ever noticed the sigh of relief that comes when you finally begin something new? After hours of labor, I let out a great sigh of relief when I looked at my newborn son cradled in my arms. Watching my son drive off for the very first time, I slowly relaxed as he began his new driving experience. I sat in the leather seats and drank in that new car smell, as I buckled the seat belt and began a wonderful relationship with my new red Honda, affectionately named "Her Honda Highness." All of these memories are new things that started with a sigh of relief.

"Relief from what?" you may ask. Everything new is preceded with pain in some degree or another. I experienced nine months of growing discomfort and eight hours of labor pains before I could begin the new experience of parenting. High anxiety preceded my son's earning his driver's license. Even now as I recall the first time I rode with my son as he drove, I tense up from my neck all the way down my spine! The old red Caravan was on its last leg before trading it in for the new Honda. The Caravan's last year was spent more in mechanics' garages than in our own garage. The sigh we experience at a new beginning is a result of being relieved from the journey through a desert or wasteland of pain that brought us to this new threshold experience.

Whenever someone finally gets it and begins to lose weight on the Live-It, I am compelled to ask, "What was it that helped you get serious about starting?" Usually they respond with, "I just couldn't stand being like *that* anymore!" It reminds me that the key to success in any new endeavor is that the motivation to change must be stronger than the desire to remain the same. In other words, we must not continue to look back at what was but rather focus on the new thing God wants to do in our life now and in the future.

Are you in a painful, hard or difficult place? If you answered yes, then things are looking up! One of two things is about to take place. You are either at the point that the pain of staying the same is becoming greater than the pain of change, or you are in the process of changing. Either way, God is about to do something new to bring you out of the wasteland and into a whole new way of living!

Nancy Taylor

What are some of your painful desert experiences? What new thing did God do to bring you out of the wasteland? Write out a prayer of thanksgiving for all the new things God has done in the past and for all that He will do in this coming year.

Lord, thank You that You are doing something new in my life. Help me to quit looking back and to focus on the new experiences You are bringing my way in this new year.

_____

_____

_____

_____

_____

_____

_____

_____

_____

_____

_____

_____

_____

_____

_____

_____

_____

_____

_____

_____

_____

_____

Forget the former things; do not dwell on the past.
See, I am doing a new thing! Now it springs up; do you not perceive it?
I am making a way in the desert and streams in the wasteland.
ISAIAH 43:18-19

Spring Forward

POPPING UP AND POOPING OUT

Forget the former things; do not dwell on the past.
See, I am doing a new thing! Now it springs up; do you not perceive it?
I am making a way in the desert and streams in the wasteland.
ISAIAH 43:18-19

It is the beginning of a new year. New Year's resolutions are popping up and pooping out. Why can't we make up our minds and stick to it? Could it be that we resolve to do new things, but we would like for them to evolve the same way we have done them in the past? We want to do new things the old way. Lose weight? Yes, but we want to do it the way we have always done it. Do you not know that God would like to do what you want Him to do, but He would like to do it in a new way?

I love the quote "God can't drive a parked car." Some of us have parked our minds in the old mode, and we cannot be moved. Can you not see that God wants to bring changes into your life if you will just shift your mind into drive and get going with God on a new street?

This past weekend I saw what would have happened in my own life if I had not shifted into drive and let God drive my car. All of the years I spent sitting in my Lazy-Boy recliner I was sitting in the desert. My life was dry and going nowhere. Through the First Place program of exercise, Bible study and Scripture memory, I sprang up out of that recliner, got out into God's world and really began to experience life.

At a 5K run, as I was walking back from the locker room, someone called me over to ask a question. Then another person stopped me, and we talked and laughed. An older gentleman who went to school with my parents also stopped to talk. As one person after another stopped me, the thought ran through my mind, "Look at all of God's people I would never have known if I had remained a parked car and never gotten out of that recliner." I am so glad God let me spring up out of that desert chair and paddle my kayak down that beautiful stream through the wasteland.

My First Place members also participated in that 5K run. When I finally got back to where they were all standing at the end of the race, I looked at them, smiled and thanked God, because if He had not taken my car out of park, I would not have had any of them in my life. I am so thankful for all of my First Place friends.

Beverly Henson

Write about areas of your life you would like God to put into overdrive.

O God, thank You for knocking my car out of park. Help me to run through life in overdrive.

_____

_____

_____

_____

_____

_____

_____

_____

_____

_____

_____

_____

_____

_____

_____

_____

_____

_____

_____

_____

_____

Forget the former things; do not dwell on the past.
See, I am doing a new thing! Now it springs up; do you not perceive it?
I am making a way in the desert and streams in the wasteland.
ISAIAH 43:18-19

Spring Forward

BUILDING BLOCKS

Forget the former things; do not dwell on the past.
See, I am doing a new thing! Now it springs up; do you not perceive it?
I am making a way in the desert and streams in the wasteland.
ISAIAH 43:18-19

What a fabulous promise for each of us to focus on as we start the new year. We can allow ourselves to become very discouraged and often depressed by dwelling on past failures. This may be the first time or the twentieth that you have allowed God to be a part of your attempt to lose weight. Success can be assured if you have faith in His promises. When you give God control of your life, He will do a new thing.

Reflect back for a minute on the life of King David and his son, Solomon. David was in battle most of his life, but his son had a different mission. Solomon was to build the temple for people to come and worship where God dwelt. We are in temple maintenance here. If you have asked Christ to be your Savior, the Holy Spirit dwells in you, and it is very important to God that this dwelling be brought up to code.

"You know that because of the wars waged against my father David from all sides, he could not build a temple for the Name of the LORD his God until the LORD put his enemies under his feet. But now the LORD my God has given me rest on every side, and there is no adversary or disaster" (1 Kings 5:3-4). Wow! Have you ever even thought to ask God to give you peace so you can work on His temple? I have thought hundreds of times how much I agree with every commitment in First Place, but life is in such turmoil, I have no time to work on myself. Here is the secret: Ask for God's peace!

I am not promising you that all of life's challenges will go away, but with each crisis that comes in our life, we really have a choice to let it stop us or let it fuel us to be more faithful. I believe that, with God's help, we can allow every brick that life throws at us to become a building block to a strong and healthy temple in which God can dwell.

Many times our defeat comes as a result of our own laziness; but if we neglect to keep our First Place commitments because life has become so difficult that we do not have time to eat healthy, have a quiet time or exercise, then it is time to stop and pray for God to give us the same peace that He gave Solomon. We are into temple maintenance here, and it is important to God.

Kay Smith

List anything in your past that comes to mind that you would consider a failure. Confess your part in that situation. Ask for God's forgiveness. List the areas of commitment or situations for which you need God's power to accomplish a miracle.

Heavenly Father, I praise You today for Your unlimited power to take my focus off the things of the past. Give me spiritual eyes to see a new thing. Father, I pray today for peace in the midst of my circumstances. I pray for Your power to use my daily trials to fuel me and not defeat me. Thank You now for doing this new thing in me.

_____
_____
_____
_____
_____
_____
_____
_____
_____
_____
_____
_____
_____
_____
_____
_____

Forget the former things; do not dwell on the past.
See, I am doing a new thing! Now it springs up; do you not perceive it?
I am making a way in the desert and streams in the wasteland.
Isaiah 43:18-19

Spring Forward

NEW BEGINNINGS

Forget the former things; do not dwell on the past.
See, I am doing a new thing! Now it springs up; do you not perceive it?
I am making a way in the desert and streams in the wasteland.
ISAIAH 43:18-19

How I love new beginnings! I love the first day of the month, week and even the early hours of each new day. I love the new moon and the full moon. I love new seasons, new leaves and new clothes!

Isn't our God wonderful for giving us a new beginning every 24 hours? If you need it broken down even further, each meal is a new beginning. If you mess up on lunch, you have a fresh do-over opportunity at dinner. If you did not exercise today, tomorrow is a new day with brand new opportunities.

This week's key verse tells us that the past is just that—past—and that we are not to dwell on it. We are not to dwell on past failures, a marriage that ended in divorce or a diet that ended in defeat. We are not to dwell on the past—period! Neither are we to dwell on past victories. Many times when I ask others what God is doing in their life, they will tell me about the time they accepted Christ 25 years ago! Our God is a God of new beginnings, and He desires to be doing something new in our lives every minute of every day. Look for it, expect it, ask for it.

A couple of years ago I had a surprising new beginning. I was in California with Jeannie Blocher, President of Body & Soul Ministries. We were there for meetings about the aerobic DVDs we wanted to partner into reality. Jeannie and I went out for a walk and as soon as we walked out of the gate where we were staying, Jeannie said, "Why don't we pray while we walk." Not wanting to look like I had never done this, I said, "Great." Jeannie started to pray, with her eyes open, I might add, walking down the sidewalk in Ventura. After a while, she stopped and I started to pray. After one glorious hour, we arrived back at our starting point to shower and dress for the day.

How do you think our meetings went that day? You guessed it, perfect in every way. The aerobic DVDs are a reality, but that's not where the story ends. Many of you know that I drive 46 miles to work every day. Well, I started doing this new thing I learned from Jeannie while driving to work! Just this week, I was so caught up in praying out loud that I missed my turn and came to work a different way than usual!

God wants to do a new thing in your life this year. Do you not perceive it?

Carole Lewis

Why not do some dreaming with God today? Write some things that you would like to begin again in this new year. Pour your heart out in confession of your past failures, asking God to forgive you. Then forget about it and begin again. This year you can do great things for God and God can do great things through you. Carpe Diem!

Dear Lord, help me in this new year to forget my past failures and not to dwell on past victories. Give me new beginnings physically, mentally, emotionally and spiritually.

Forget the former things; do not dwell on the past.
See, I am doing a new thing! Now it springs up; do you not perceive it?
I am making a way in the desert and streams in the wasteland.
ISAIAH 43:18-19

Spring Forward

WHAT'S UP?

Forget the former things; do not dwell on the past.
See, I am doing a new thing! Now it springs up; do you not perceive it?
I am making a way in the desert and streams in the wasteland.
ISAIAH 43:18-19

"What's up?" is a greeting I often hear exchanged between today's young people. Translation: "What are you up to these days?" This is a great question! However, most people ask it rhetorically, not expecting a real answer. We do the same with God. We ask Him what in the world He is doing now, but often do not stick around for the answer!

One of the most congested freeway interchanges in the entire country is located right outside our office door! For years people have experienced the headache and hassle of traffic jams on the Katy Freeway in Houston. Finally, the freeway is being expanded to allow for more traffic flow. Each day as we travel to work, we ask each other about the construction. We try to speculate on how all these new roads are going to meet. It looks like a bowlful of spaghetti—so many twists and turns with no end in sight! We are always questioning how in the world it is all going to work. Since we travel these roads daily we are very observant of what has been done each day. We can see when a lane is opened or when a bridge has been torn down or a railing added to a new bridge. We even had a little celebration for the construction workers when a lane was opened by inviting them in for refreshments.

As we embark on a new year, let's be more observant. Take time daily as you travel through God's Word to ask Him, "What's up?" Look to see how He is providing a new road for you to travel or a path leading out of a rough situation you have encountered. You may be questioning whether you will be able to meet those weight-loss goals or to read the Bible through this year. Instead of questioning yourself, ask God what He is doing. His answer will be "See, I am doing something new! Now it springs up; do you not perceive it? I am making a way in the desert and streams in the wasteland." Then, celebrate the new things He does all through the year.

Nancy Taylor

Look for God today. List all the ways God worked in your life yesterday and today. Ask Him what He is up to in your life and then watch and listen to see if you can perceive the new work He is doing on your behalf.

Lord, help me to be more observant of what You are doing in my life. Thank You that You are doing something new and that You will provide new roadways for me to travel and new ways to help me reach my goals.

Forget the former things; do not dwell on the past.
See, I am doing a new thing! Now it springs up; do you not perceive it?
I am making a way in the desert and streams in the wasteland.
ISAIAH 43:18-19

New Creation

NEW WARDROBE

Therefore, if anyone is in Christ, he is a new creation;
the old has gone, the new has come!
2 CORINTHIANS 5:17

One of my favorite Bible stories is the story of Joseph. I particularly like the part when Pharaoh sent for him at the prison in which he was being held. He was cleaned up, shaved and presented as a new person to stand before the king. It was a new day for Joseph. For many of us in First Place, God would like to give us a new day at the beginning of this new year. He would like for us to throw away our prison clothes and look at the world through new-creation eyes.

Most of my adult life I was going up and down the scales like a yo-yo on a string. I had a closet full of clothes in all sizes to reflect my trips up and down the scales. Some were really big, some really small and some in every size in between, just in case I might need them. I now call them my prison clothes. As long as I had them to fall back on, I could gain weight or lose it and always have clothes to accommodate me no matter my size. By holding on to those clothes I was holding myself in prison. The day I got rid of them was the day I truly stepped out of the prison in which I was being held.

If anyone is in Christ, He is a new creation. A new creation in Jesus sees the world through new eyes. She looks for new thoughts and new ideas to keep her out of prison. New creations, who were bought with a price by their King Jesus, think like their King. They can say, "I am a new creature in Jesus Christ; He has freed me from the food prison in which I have been living. I am free, so I don't need these old clothes anymore."

The old has gone; the new has come. We have to remove the old things before the new can take their rightful place. Take pride in the fact that you are a new creation. Do a bit of housecleaning. Get the old stuff out to the curb for trash pickup. We have new stuff coming. Jesus has a new wardrobe for you!

Beverly Henson

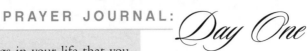
List the things in your life that you need to take to the curbside for trash pickup to make way for the new things God wants to do with your life.

Thank You, Father, for clothing me with new thoughts and ideas.

_____

_____

_____

_____

_____

_____

_____

_____

_____

_____

_____

_____

_____

_____

_____

_____

_____

_____

_____

Therefore, if anyone is in Christ, he is a new creation;
the old has gone, the new has come!
2 CORINTHIANS 5:17

New Creation

STYLIN'!

*Therefore, if anyone is in Christ, he is a new creation;
the old has gone, the new has come!*
2 CORINTHIANS 5:17

When I was growing up, my mom sewed all my clothes. I took this blessing entirely for granted, thinking that every child was as fortunate as I was. The times that we purchased clothing for me to wear were so few and far between that I remember each one as a special occasion.

It was nothing for me to come home from school on Friday afternoon to find that a brand-new dress had been created for me to wear to a party that night. When it was prom time, my mom drove me to the most expensive dress shop in town. I tried on beautiful, expensive dresses until I settled on the one I wanted. My mom then took out her notepad and began taking notes: 1-inch wide ruffles, ribbon on the edge of each ruffle, etc.

After we returned from the store, she duplicated the beautiful dress I had tried on, and on prom night, no one was the wiser. I was in a new creation that was considerably cheaper to make at home than to purchase.

The one thing I never gave a thought to was what it cost my mom in time and energy to give me my new gown. The same is true spiritually. It took Jesus' shed blood on the cross so that you and I might wear our new clothes of righteousness.

This week's verse explains what it means to be a new creation in Christ. Our old tattered rags of sin are gone—every last one of them forgiven by the shed blood of Christ. We are now dressed in the righteousness of Christ every day. The old ways are gone, and old habits are replaced with new ones that look like a million bucks, inside and out! As the kids say, "We're stylin'!"

This year, every day is an opportunity to look beautiful in our new clothes of compassion, kindness, humility, gentleness and patience. Need something new? Ask Jesus; He's the master tailor!

Carole Lewis

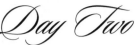
Write a letter to God. Praise Him for the miracle of making you a new creation in Christ. Confess to Him your sorrow over not wearing the new beautiful clothes created especially for you. Thank Him that you no longer have to wear your rags of sin. Write about the progress you have seen this last year in your Christian walk. Write about the progress you desire to achieve this new year.

Dear Lord, I know that I am a new creation in Christ so why am I content to wear the old tattered rags of the past?

Clothe me in Your grace and mercy this year. Cleanse my heart of all the old things that drag me down, and show me what it means to live as a new creation.

_____

_____

_____

_____

_____

_____

_____

_____

_____

_____

_____

_____

_____

_____

_____

_____

_____

_____

_____

Therefore, if anyone is in Christ, he is a new creation;
the old has gone, the new has come!
2 CORINTHIANS 5:17

New Creation

NEW BEGINNING

Therefore, if anyone is in Christ, he is a new creation;
the old has gone, the new has come!
2 CORINTHIANS 5:17

I thank God that He is a God of new beginnings. I accepted Christ as my Savior at a very young age and remember telling my mom that I was a new person. I also remember her reminding me of that statement two days later when I had been ugly to my younger sister. Well, that was my first lesson in beginning again. I learned just two days into being a new creation that my soul was saved but that I have this fleshly desire to have what I want when I want it. I asked God to forgive me—which He did—and I began again.

My First Place journey has also given me plenty of opportunities to tell God just how sorry I am that I have not been as obedient as I should be, and that I would appreciate a new beginning. He has forgiven me, and we begin again. I have found First Place to be a very self-motivating program but often talk to leaders and members who are struggling. They are usually looking for something new to motivate them. My answer is always the same. Through past experience I have found that I do not need to learn something new but that I need a new beginning to do the right things. The key is to get back to the basics. I go over the nine commitments, confess to God what I am not doing and ask for His strength to do each one for just one day. I do exactly the same thing the second day, and usually by the third day, I am thinking, *What was so hard about this?*

First Place is a program that you cannot fail. You may experience lapses, and even relapses, but what you want to avoid is a collapse. I have a three-part plan that guarantees success: The first is your part—the work. You may need to buy good tennis shoes; purge your kitchen of unhealthy food choices; plan healthy meals; fill the kitchen with good food choices; or arrange your Bible, Bible Study and prayer journal in a special spot for quiet time. The second is God's part—the strength. Be honest with God about where you need His strength and be ready to step out in faith. The third is the part of others—to support. Reach out to others in your group; tell them exactly what you are struggling with and ask for prayer. You may need a friend to exercise with, or you may need to meet with an alumni member to help you understand the Live-It. You are also given a chance to support others. Look for those opportunities.

Expecting the leader or other members to do your work or give you strength will only lead to problems. Thinking that the leader or any member should be responsible for the work—your part—will only lead to frustration. God is the only source of strength you will need. You are the only one who can do this work. Accept the support of your team members. You will succeed.

Kay Smith

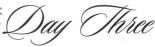

List each commitment that you are not completing. Get very specific about what you need to do to get started or to complete this commitment. Write down how your class members could support you better. List any thoughts you have about supporting others in your class.

Heavenly Father, I thank You for the power that You have made available to me. I ask You today to forgive me in all areas in which I have not been doing my part. I ask for Your strength as I take a step of faith to be faithful in each of the areas. I pray for You to give me the strength to be vulnerable in my prayer request and accept the support of my team members. I pray for You to enlighten me to any situations in this group for which I could offer my support.

_____

_____

_____

_____

_____

_____

_____

_____

_____

_____

_____

_____

_____

*Therefore, if anyone is in Christ, he is a new creation;
the old has gone, the new has come!*
2 Corinthians 5:17

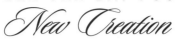
New Creation

PAST DELETED

Therefore, if anyone is in Christ, he is a new creation;
the old has gone, the new has come!
2 CORINTHIANS 5:17

As much as I love the Christmas season and the beautifully decorated Christmas trees, on the day after Christmas the tree suddenly becomes stark and barren. All the presents are gone, the mystery of the contents has been revealed, and the magic of the previous day is gone. My thoughts immediately move to putting away all the decorations, cleaning and restoring the house, and looking toward a brand-new year waiting just around the corner.

How depressing it would be to leave the Christmas trappings in our house all year long, while throughout the new year we tried to recapture the magic of the Christmas past. What if our days were consumed with thoughts about gifts we should have bought, meals we could have prepared differently, and calories we should not have consumed? The new year would come and go, but we would be unable to enjoy God's blessings because we would still be dwelling on the past.

For those of you with home computers, have you ever unintentionally hit the delete button and your screen suddenly went blank? I certainly have, more times than I care to remember. No matter how you try to retrieve the information, it is forever gone. What a blessing that when we become a member of God's household, we are a new creation. Our past has been deleted and becomes a blank screen, ready to be filled with new things.

Isaiah 43:18-19 says, "Forget the former things; do not dwell on the past. See, I am doing a new thing." We cannot go forward as long as we are looking backward. God has new and wonderful things for us this year. Hit the delete button on your past and eagerly watch to see what new things God has planned for you this new year.

Pat Lewis

Is there any old thing in your past you would like deleted? Confess it to God and accept His forgiveness. He will hit His delete button, and you will have a blank screen before Him once again.

Father, how we thank You that when we give our lives to You, our past is a blank screen. You forgive all our sins and give us a new abundant life with joy and peace everlasting. Your mercies are new every morning.

_____

_____

_____

_____

_____

_____

_____

_____

_____

_____

_____

_____

_____

_____

_____

_____

_____

Therefore, if anyone is in Christ, he is a new creation;
the old has gone, the new has come!
2 CORINTHIANS 5:17

New Creation

SOME ASSEMBLY REQUIRED!

*Therefore, if anyone is in Christ, he is a new creation;
the old has gone, the new has come!*
2 CORINTHIANS 5:17

Have you ever had one of those days? You know the kind I am talking about—nothing seems to come easy and you are faced with one challenge after another. This past Saturday was one of those days for me. It had been two weeks since I had cleaned my house, and I scheduled the entire day for dusting, vacuuming, cleaning bathrooms and getting some holiday decorating done. An hour into my schedule, I began the task of vacuuming in hopes of removing all the black dog hair that had accumulated. As I was vacuuming, I noticed that the hair was only being redistributed throughout the living room. Soon it became evident that the vacuum cleaner had seen its last day of work! I made a quick phone call to my husband, who was running some errands for me, and let him know the bad news. He said he would buy a new vacuum cleaner and be home as soon as he could. About an hour later, my husband appeared with a new vacuum cleaner, unassembled, of course!

I waded through the ambiguous assembly instructions with anxious anticipation of my new creation! In my rush to put the machine together, I found myself pushing when I was supposed to be pulling and shoving instead of sliding. Then I realized that if I not only looked at the pictures but also read the instructions, the assembly actually went rather smoothly! Finally, I was able to vacuum my carpet with great efficiency, even though I was now about two hours behind schedule!

I am always so excited to see the first day of January arrive each year. It marks a new beginning, a fresh start and hopefully a new me! I can get so caught up in dreams and visions of my new year with new opportunities that I forget to stop and read the instructions. First, God's Word tells us that if we are *in Christ*, we are new creatures. Every day we are new! We don't need to wait until a new year to celebrate the *new*, because when we accept the gift of salvation, we also get another free gift—a new life! Second, the Word says that the old is gone and the new has come. I was so glad to throw out that old, broken vacuum cleaner and begin with a new one! When we hang on to the old, we lose some precious time by trying to redistribute our old life into our new one. That doesn't work! Instead, we must take on a new way of thinking and a new way of acting.

To assemble this new life God has given, you must take in His Word daily, reading the instructions for life and following those instructions by doing what they say.

Nancy Taylor

Day Five

What are some old thoughts and actions that still mark your life? Write those in your journal, and ask the Lord to teach you His truth concerning these thoughts and actions.

Lord, thank You for the gift of a new life that is only found in Christ. Lord, open my eyes each day that I may receive instructions from Your Word and truly live as a new creation in Christ.

_____

_____

_____

_____

_____

_____

_____

_____

_____

_____

_____

_____

_____

_____

_____

_____

_____

_____

_____

Therefore, if anyone is in Christ, he is a new creation;
the old has gone, the new has come!
2 CORINTHIANS 5:17

New Creation

BRAND-NEW AND BEAUTIFUL

Therefore, if anyone is in Christ, he is a new creation;
the old has gone, the new has come!
2 CORINTHIANS 5:17

I came to Christ when I was 12 years old. At that age I hadn't done any heavy-duty sinning. Sure, I had disobeyed my parents, but I hadn't even begun to know how rotten sin really looks in the life of an unbeliever. It looks even more rotten in the life of a believer!

I don't get as excited about a new car as my husband does. In fact, for years I had never had a new car. Johnny needed the good car for work so I drove one clunker after another. A friend and I used to joke that we would take whichever one of our cars was running that day to run an errand at lunch!

About 10 years ago, when I finally got my first new car, I absolutely loved it. The new-car smell is so wonderful that they even have a new-car smell at the car wash! The upholstery didn't have one stain on it. The floor mats were fresh and new. There were no empty wrappers strewn about and all the storage compartments were empty!

Each of us has the ability to look and feel like that new car every minute of every day. As believers, all we need to do is confess our sin when we commit it, instead of letting our sin pile up until a marathon cleaning is necessary. When our kids were small, our car would get so piled up with litter that each of us would have to carry an armload of trash into the house from the car.

God designed us so that we can stay clean and new all the time; it's our choice. "The new has come" means that after we accept Jesus personally into our life, we have the very power of God residing inside of us. "The old has gone, the new has come!"

Celebrate the new creation that you are in Christ today. Clean up your temple, and keep it clean this year. If you do, you'll keep that new-car look and smell all year long!

Carole Lewis

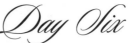
Talk to God about what it means to be a new creation in Christ. Confess the old things that you desire to be rid of and claim your new start with Him. Ask Him to keep reminding you that "the old has gone, the new has come!"

Dear Father, Help me this year to take care of my temple like I would a fancy new car. Help me keep it clean, inside and out. Forgive me for abusing Your creation and help me make a fresh start.

Therefore, if anyone is in Christ, he is a new creation;
the old has gone, the new has come!
2 CORINTHIANS 5:17

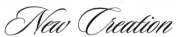

New Creation

STAYING CURRENT

Therefore, if anyone is in Christ, he is a new creation;
the old has gone, the new has come!
2 Corinthians 5:17

I served the Lord as a children's pastor for almost 10 years. During that time, puppet ministries were very popular with the children. One of the neatest series of music we used with our puppets was Psalty, a singing songbook. The music was really cute and the kids just loved it. There were songs titled "Sandyland," "Heaven Is a Wonderful Place" and "The Wa-Wa Song." It was great, but those children grew up and a new group of children came. They thought Psalty was nerdy and they didn't like it. I became angry because Psalty was cute, and I loved it. One Sunday I told them that Psalty was what we were using and that they needed to learn to like it. But they didn't like it, and I couldn't make them.

The Lord really dealt with me through this time about staying current. He told me I needed to be open to new things. I prayed about it, then went out and bought a few Christian rap tunes. I won the hearts of those kids, and children's church was a rocking place to be once again. Sometimes we try to hang on to our Psaltys long after we should let them go. When we do this, we don't even notice when God is doing a new thing.

In First Place, as we become successful with our weight loss, we become comfortable at times with the way we did it when we first started. I have had my weight off for over five years now and constantly have to change my exercise and food intake to maintain the level of fitness I strive to achieve. Many times we find that as we go down in weight, we have to stop something we are eating that is okay and begin to do a new thing.

We have to stay in tune with the Lord. He is the best personal trainer I know. He will help us stay current with our new body tunes even when we try to keep the old Psalty on the scene. We are a new creation in Him. New creations walk to the beat of new songs. Strive to stay current.

Beverly Henson

List the areas in your life in which you feel you have become stale and for which you would like the Lord to give you current upgrades.

Father, help me stay current with the things You need to do in my life.

Therefore, if anyone is in Christ, he is a new creation;
the old has gone, the new has come!
2 CORINTHIANS 5:17

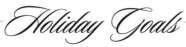

Holiday Goals

"Commit to the Lord whatever you do, and your plans will succeed."
PROVERBS 16:3

During the Thanksgiving and Christmas holidays, many temptations will come our way. It will become more and more difficult to remain faithful to the Nine Commitments as we are bombarded with activities that will demand our time and attention. That is why we need a PLAN! The plan is to commit to the Lord your desire to reach your First Place goals and to remain consistent in practicing the spiritual and physical disciplines you have already begun. Remember, this is a lifetime journey, and one wrong turn doesn't mean the journey is over! So one poor food choice or one missed quiet time doesn't give us permission to give up. We must plan to succeed, and when we fail, we must plan to begin again! Develop strategies that will help you be successful during the holidays.

MY GOALS FOR THE HOLIDAY SEASON

1. _____

2. _____

3. _____

STRATEGIES TO HELP ME BE SUCCESSFUL IN THESE GOALS

EXERCISE PLANS

1. _____

2. _____

3. _____

HOLIDAY HELPS: WELLNESS WORKSHEET ONE

LIVE-IT STRATEGIES

1. _____

2. _____

3. _____

PLANS FOR SPIRITUAL HEALTH

1. _____

2. _____

3. _____

STRESS MANAGEMENT

1. _____

2. _____

3. _____

No-Worry Thanksgiving!

- Before the big day, experiment with recipes to familiarize yourself with their preparation. Get everything out on the counter ready to go.
- Prepare as much as possible in advance. For example: Homemade cranberry sauce tastes better after curing in the refrigerator for a few days; premeasure seasonings, and store them in labeled bags or containers; clean, cut and store vegetables in plastic bags in the refrigerator.
- Let your family set the table. Children will gobble up the chance to make place cards, fold napkins, and dress up the holiday table. This will also keep them out of the kitchen while you attend to the food.
- Serve buffet style. With pretty serving bowls and silver utensils guests can help themselves to seconds whenever they want, while you remember your portion sizes.
- Let the turkey rest before slicing. To avoid a last-minute crunch and assure tender turkey, let the bird rest out of the oven, covered, for about 30 minutes before slicing.
- Use your microwave oven. Take advantage of this appliance to quickly reheat food before serving when all the burners on the stovetop are occupied.
- Thermometers are essential for food safety. When choosing a meat thermometer, look for an easy-to-read dial with a stainless-steel face and shatterproof lens. Check the thermometer for accuracy by submerging at least two inches of the stem in boiling water. It should read 212 degrees F (or the boiling temperature of water at your altitude). An alternative to the typical meat thermometer is an instant-read thermometer, also known as a rapid-response thermometer, which is designed to measure a wide range of temperatures, typically from 0 degrees F to 220 degrees F. It does not stay in food during cooking. When it's inserted in the food, the temperature should register in about 15 seconds.
- Finally, remember that this is Thanksgiving. Take time to thank God for what He has done in your life this past year and for what He is going to do for you in the coming year.

Bon Appétit!
Scott Wilson
Jeremiah 29:11

Holiday Survival Tips

Maintaining healthy eating habits and an exercise regimen during the holidays can seem like an overwhelming task. Many times all of our good habits that we have worked so hard to develop are thrown out the window as soon as November arrives! Planning ahead for holiday challenges is the key to surviving the holidays with those healthy habits intact. Following these weekly suggestions will help you experience a healthier holiday season:

WEEK ONE: FOCUS

- Find a holiday exercise buddy to walk with you daily or attend an aerobics class together. Make exercise a priority!
- Find healthy holiday recipes that will fit into the Live-It and ones that you will enjoy serving to holiday visitors.
- Focus on friends and family rather than on food. Make a special gift for each person attending your holiday get-together. Take Polaroid (or digital) group pictures and place in a Thanksgiving card for each person to take home with him or her as a keepsake.

WEEK TWO: SHOPPING SAVVY

- Park far away from the front door of the mall! Walk briskly, get some exercise, and save time looking for parking places.
- Stop in the name of health! Don't even think of stopping for a treat at the food court! Pack some shopping snacks in your bag: yogurt, raisins, an apple, a banana or pretzels. This will prove to be a money saver and a calorie cutter.
- Warm up. Before actually making any purchases, take a stroll through the entire mall, then go back to make purchases. This will not only add steps to your shopping day, but also will help you make informed decisions about your purchases.

WEEK THREE: HEALTHY ACTIVITIES

- Start a neighborhood tradition. Invite your neighbors to walk the neighborhood or community and sing Christmas carols along the way.

- Volunteer to help a young mom by taking her young child for a stroller ride.
- Help out at a soup kitchen, or clean out your closets and donate the items to a local charity.

WEEK FOUR: PARTY HEARTY
Holiday parties can sabotage your healthy eating plan, but with a little planning you can enjoy them without overindulging.

- Avoid the buffet table. Find someone to visit with who is sitting far away from the food. Focus on conversation, not eating.
- Keep a glass of water or diet soda in your hands. This will keep one fewer hand out of the high calorie goodies.
- Bring a healthy appetizer like raw veggies or fruit to ensure that you will have something to snack on that will support your healthy habits.

WEEK FIVE: THE PARTY'S OVER
- If you end up with leftovers that are tempting, send them home with your guests or share them with an elderly friend or a family.
- Freeze some of the leftovers in single servings to take for lunches or to have for dinners on the run.
- In preparation for the new year, purge your pantry of any junk foods or tempting foods. Out with the old, in with the new!

WEEK SIX: A NEW BEGINNING
- Greet the new year with a healthy attitude. Write one goal for the year in each of these areas: spiritual, emotional, mental and physical.
- Start the new year off by planning your first week of menus along with your shopping list.
- Renew any health newsletters or magazines for the coming year, or sign up to receive free health and fitness e-mail newsletters or other publications.

And let us consider how we may spur one another on toward love and good deeds.
HEBREWS 10:24

*Jesus looked at them and said, "With man this is impossible,
but with God all things are possible."*
MATTHEW 19:26

Dear Family,

I have thought about our Christmas this year and wondered what would give it more fullness. It seems that when we help someone else, we gain pleasure and satisfaction and become better people. Our happiness is not always just a result of getting something. We all have so very many good things. Could we share our gifts this year with others?

This year, I am challenging you—***should you choose to accept this mission***—to take the enclosed Christmas check and decide how best to use it.

After considering the possibilities, you may

- Buy something for yourself.
- Use a portion of it to buy yourself what you want and the other portion to share with another person who has less or needs help.
- Work together with other family members to complete a project.

When we get together for Christmas, please bring all of your gifts to open that day. Wrap the gift for yourself. Wrap the gift that you are sharing with someone else. If you have already given them the gift, put something in the box that tells the story of your gift to share with the rest of us.

I love you all and look forward to a special time together at Christmas this year.

Blessings,

PS: Some ideas
1. Volunteer to serve a holiday meal to needy families.

2. Give a gift to someone in another country through Heifer International or Samaritan's Purse. Check out their websites:
   www.heifer.org
   www.samaritanspurse.org
3. Send cards to military service personnel. Access www.anysoldier.com for further information.
4. American Legion takes gift donations for American soldiers who get few letters and gifts and are serving in other countries.
5. Give donations to a food pantry.
6. Find a project in your church or community.
7. Donate time and/or gifts to a nonprofit group.

Healthy Holiday Cooking Hints

- Purchase a turkey without added fat; i.e., those that have butter or oil injected under the skin.
- If you use broth from the turkey, remove the fat. This can be done by allowing the broth to cool in the refrigerator or by using ice cubes to remove the fat.
- Pies are a great holiday dessert. Quick and easy pies can be made from instant or cook-and-serve sugar-free pudding. Any flavor fruit pie can be made by using fresh fruit such as apples or peaches. Slice fruit, place in a saucepan, add a cup of apple juice or other fruit juice and one cup of water; cook until softened. Sweeten to taste with artificial sweetener. Add spices, if desired, and thicken with cornstarch. You now have a sugar-free, fat-free filling. See the *New First Place Favorites* recipe book for more great pies.
- Applesauce is a great substitute for fat and sugar in recipes. You can exchange a half cup of applesauce for a half cup of oil. Or a half cup of an artificial sweetener can be exchanged for a half cup of the sugar. The chart for these equivalents is listed in the *New First Place Favorites* recipe book. **Note:** Substantial amounts of substitutes for the sugar and oil do not exchange well. That is why it is best to only replace part of the sugar or oil.
- The holiday season is a good time to experiment with dips. Use plain yogurt instead of sour cream. Even though the fat-free sour cream is devoid of fat grams, it is also devoid of nutrients. Keep in mind that our goal in First Place is to eat foods with as many nutrients as possible.
- Add yogurt mixed with fruit to Jell-O for a creamy dessert.

Bring Joy to the Season

- Send Christmas notes to at least six people who blessed you this past year. For example: Thank your First Place leader or a member who has encouraged you. Be specific about how they helped you.
- Call someone who may be having a sad holiday and let them know you are thinking of them. For example: a friend who had a death in the family during the year or someone who is ill.
- Invite someone to be a part of your holiday celebration who would have little family activity otherwise. For example: Take that person to a church party or to look at Christmas lights.
- Make a spiritual event part of your Christmas tradition. For example: Read the Christmas story in Matthew 1:18-25; Luke 2:1-20 and Matthew 2:1-12; attend a candlelight service or a church pageant.
- Tell stories of family Christmases past. Find visual reminders such as old decorations, cards, photos or gifts of past Christmases that you have experienced. Share stories that older relatives have told about their Christmases. Heirloom stories tie families to their heritage and encourage them to make memories for the future.
- Mail new year's greetings to as many friends and family as possible. The time after Christmas is often a period when you can have more time to be reflective and the notes are not lost in all the Christmas mail.
- SLOW DOWN, take a deep breath and plan a successful and meaningful holiday.
- DROP the unimportant, even if others want to pressure you.
- ADD the important, even if no one but you finds meaning in it.
- ENJOY people more than things and the gift of the Son of God more than anything else!

When He is first place, *all the season's events hold the potential for JOY.*

Emotional Traps

- *Comparison.* Festive outings can be occasions for being placed in uncomfortable situations that give rise to feelings of inferiority, embarrassment or shame. This may occur at company dinners, family gatherings or church parties where poise and physical appearance seem to be more important than ever. These situations may stir up past feelings of not measuring up that can date back to a childhood party or an embarrassing blunder in a Christmas play.
- *Expectations.* For many people, the holidays are not emotional lifts, instead they are emotional downers. They make tough times seem tougher and sad times seem sadder because of the expectations that this is to be the happiest time of the year and that everyone else is full of joy. Sometimes we have idealized expectations for holiday events that are not based in reality, and when those expectations are not met, we might become depressed. Learn to be realistic about your expectations.
- *Difficult Settings.* Perhaps unlike any other time of the year, the time between Thanksgiving and New Year's Day draws more families together than at any other time. If family gatherings are affirming, they can be a wonderfully emotional time. But for millions of people, the holidays are filled with past pain, guilt, unresolved anger, destructive secrets and old unhealthy patterns.

  Examples of painful family situations can be a divorced couple splitting Christmas with the children, or an adult visiting an overcontrolling mother, an abusive alcoholic father or an out-of-control, drug-abusing sibling. In order to minimize the negative influence of holiday distractions to healthy living, it is important to increase the positive factors.
- *Evaluate.* Looking over the past few holiday seasons, consider what caused pain and what caused joy. Add more of the joy factors (e.g., sponsor a needy family or attend a Christmas Eve service). Attempt to discover patterns of pain, and make plans to minimize their impact before they occur (e.g., keep your visit short or put off a visit until a less stressful time).
- *Support.* Seek the support of at least two people to be your reality check and prayer-support partners. They can give their impression of what is a rea-

sonable or healthy reaction to low self-esteem issues or painful family situations.

- *Plan.* Don't just let the holidays sweep you along. Plan now what you will or won't do.

Holiday Menus and Recipes

EACH PLAN IS BASED ON APPROXIMATELY 1,400 CALORIES.

Breakfast	0-1 meat, 1-2 breads, 1 fruit, 0-1 milk, 0-½ fat
Lunch	2 meats, 2 breads, 1 vegetable, 1 fruit, 1 fat
Dinner	3 meats, 2 breads, 2 vegetables, 1 fat
Snacks	1 bread, 1 fruit, 1 milk, ½-1 fat (or any remaining exchanges)

FOR MORE CALORIES, ADD THE FOLLOWING TO THE 1,400-CALORIE PLAN:

1,600 calories	2 breads, 1 fat
1,800 calories	2 meats, 3 breads, 1 vegetable, 1 fat
2,000 calories	2 meats, 4 breads, 1 vegetable, 3 fats
2,200 calories	2 meats, 5 breads, 1 vegetable, 1 fruit, 5 fats
2,400 calories	2 meats, 6 breads, 2 vegetables, 1 fruit, 6 fats

The exchanges for these meals were calculated using the MasterCook software. It uses a database of over 6,000 food items prepared using United States Department of Agriculture (USDA) publications and information from food manufacturers. As with any nutritional program, MasterCook calculates the nutritional values of the recipes based on ingredients. Nutrition may vary due to how the food is prepared, where the food comes from, soil content, season, ripeners, processing and methods of preparation. For these reasons, please use the recipes and menu plans as approximate guides. As always, consult your physician and/or a registered dietitian before starting a diet program.

Note: Recipes for entrees in boldface italics follow the menus.

BREAKFAST

1	c. nonfat milk
1 ¼	c. strawberries (or other fruit)
½	c. bran flake cereal

Exchanges: 1 bread, 1 fruit, 1 milk

~~~~~~

THANKSGIVING MEAL

1	4-oz. serving *Roast Turkey with Herbs*
1	c. *Crock-Pot Dressing*
2	tbsp. *Creamy Turkey Gravy*
1	c. *Green Beans and Pickled Red Onions*
½	c. *Apple Salad Mold*
1	oz. roll
⅛	slice *Easy Pumpkin Pie*

Exchanges: 3 meats, 3 ½ breads, 2 ½ vegetables, ½ fruit, ¼ milk, 2 ½ fats

~~~~~~

DINNER

(May be used for lunch or dinner)

1	turkey bagel sandwich, made with
	1 small (2 oz.) bagel
	2 oz. cooked turkey, sliced
	1 tsp. low-fat mayonnaise
	2 tomato slices and
	2 romaine lettuce leaves
1	c. carrot sticks
1	c. broccoli florets
1	tbsp. low-fat Ranch dressing
	Fresh fruit with ½-cup fat-free yogurt

Exchanges: 2 meats, 2 breads, 2 vegetables, 1 ½ fruits, ½ milk, ½ fat

~~~~~~

Total exchanges for the day: 5 meats, 6 ½ breads, 4 ½ vegetables, 3 fruits, 2 milks, 3 fats

ROAST TURKEY WITH HERBS

Serves 15 to 20

(**Note:** If you are using a frozen turkey, allow 3 to 4 days for turkey to thaw in the refrigerator; do not thaw on the kitchen counter)

¼	c. minced onion
½	tsp. dried leaf thyme
½	tsp. dried rubbed sage
3	tbsp. grated lemon rind
¼	c. chicken broth
10 to 12	lbs. turkey (completely thawed if frozen)
2	c. chicken or turkey broth
	Nonstick cooking spray

Preheat oven to 400° F. Combine first 5 ingredients (onion through broth). Remove giblets from turkey cavity and discard; rinse turkey and pat dry. Lift skin away from turkey breast and spread mixture between skin and turkey. Use any remaining herb mixture in turkey cavity. Place turkey on rack that has been sprayed with nonstick cooking spray; put rack in roasting pan and pour broth around turkey. Roast turkey at 400° F for 30 minutes. Reduce oven temperature to 350° F; continue roasting until meat thermometer inserted into thickest part of thigh registers 175° F, about 2 hours. (Baste every 30 minutes, if desired.) Transfer turkey to platter; tent with foil and let stand 30 minutes to let the juices set. Do not cut turkey for 30 minutes. Serve yourself a 4-ounce portion.

Exchanges: 4 meats

~~~~~~

CREAMY TURKEY GRAVY

Serves 12

1½	c. chicken broth (low sodium) or defatted turkey drippings
¼	c. evaporated skim milk
3	tbsp. all-purpose flour
1	tsp. melted reduced-calorie butter
½	tsp. pepper, or to taste
1	hard cooked egg, finely chopped

Heat broth in a medium saucepan over medium heat. Put next 4 ingredients in a small bowl and whisk until smooth, or put in a jar with a tight-fitting lid and shake until smooth. Gradually stir into chicken broth. Cook over medium heat for 3 to 5 minutes or until thickened, stirring constantly. Add the chopped egg. Makes about 2 cups.

Exchanges for 2 tablespoons of gravy: Free

~~~~~~

CROCK-POT DRESSING

Serves 12

12	c. day-old bread cubes
½	c. reduced-calorie butter
2	c. chopped onion
2	c. chopped celery
2	8-oz. cans sliced mushrooms
½	c. thinly sliced green onions
1	tsp. poultry seasoning
1	tsp. sage
½	tsp. pepper
¼	tsp. garlic powder
3½	c. chicken or turkey broth, defatted
2	eggs, well beaten

Place bread cubes in a very large mixing bowl. Melt butter in a skillet and sauté onion, celery and mushrooms. Pour over bread cubes. Add green onions and all seasonings and toss well. Pour in enough broth to moisten. Add eggs and mix well. Pack lightly into slow cooker. Cover and cook on low for 6 to 8 hours.

Exchanges for 1 cup of dressing: 1-½ breads, ½ vegetable, 1 fat

~~~~~~

GREEN BEANS AND PICKLED RED ONIONS

Serves 12

2	tbsp. olive oil
2	large red onions, thinly sliced
1	tsp. leaf oregano
¼	c. balsamic vinaigrette
3	lbs. fresh green beans, trimmed
	Juice of 1 lemon
	Salt and pepper to taste

Heat a large skillet over medium heat; add olive oil, sliced onion and oregano. Cook onion, stirring occasionally, until soft and translucent; add the balsamic vinaigrette. (Either keep warm and set aside or make ahead and refrigerate; heat onions before adding to green beans.) Cook green beans in a large kettle of boiling salted water. Do not cover; cook for approximately 7 minutes or until beans are brightly colored, but still a little crisp. Drain, squeeze lemon juice over beans and toss. Add salt and pepper to taste and toss with pickled onions. Serve hot.

Exchanges: 2 vegetables, 1 fat

~~~~~~

APPLE SALAD MOLD

1	3-oz. sugar-free cherry Jell-O (or any flavor)
1	c. boiling water
½	c. apple juice
½	c. cold water
1	medium unpeeled apple, chopped (about 1 ½ cups)
½	c. chopped celery

Put dry gelatin in a medium bowl. Pour in boiling water; stir for 2 minutes. Combine juice and cold water. Add to gelatin and stir. Refrigerate until slightly thickened. Add apple and celery. Mix well. Refrigerate until set. Makes five ½ cup servings.

Exchange per ½ cup serving: ½ fruit

~~~~~~

EASY PUMPKIN PIE

Serves 8

1	16-oz. can solid-packed pumpkin
1	13-oz. can evaporated skim milk
1	egg
2	egg whites
½	c. reduced-fat buttermilk biscuit mix
8	packets Sweet & Low (¾ tablespoon)
½	tsp. ground nutmeg
2	tsp. vanilla
½	tsp. ground cinnamon
½	tsp. ground ginger
	Vegetable cooking spray
	Lite Cool Whip for garnish

Place all ingredients into bowl of a food processor or blender and process until smooth. Pour into pie pan that has been coated with cooking spray. Bake at 350° F for 45-50 minutes or until center is puffed up. Let cool and put a dollop (1 teaspoon) of Cool Whip on each slice of pie.

Exchanges per $\frac{1}{8}$ pie serving: 1 bread, $\frac{1}{4}$ milk, $\frac{1}{2}$ fat

~ ~

WILD RICE AND TURKEY SALAD

Serves 4

½	c. wild rice
1½	c. water
¼	c. chopped green onions
2	tbsp. olive oil
¾	lb. cooked turkey, cut in bite-size pieces
2	tbsp. red or white wine vinegar
1	c. cherry tomatoes, cut in half
1	c. chopped celery
¼	tsp. black pepper
½	c. chopped sweet red pepper
¼	tsp. nutmeg
2	tbsp. chopped fresh parsley leaves
⅓	c. raisins
1	medium apple, chopped
1	tbsp. chopped pecans for garnish

Cook the rice in water until tender, about 50 minutes. Add green onions the last 5 minutes of cooking time. Combine all ingredients in a large bowl and toss. Cover and chill until ready to serve. Sprinkle with pecans just before serving.

Exchanges per ½-cup serving : 3 meats, ¾ bread, ¾ vegetable, 1¼ fruits, 1¾ fats

~ ~

OVEN-ROASTED SWEET POTATOES

Serves 12

5	medium-size sweet potatoes, peeled and cut into 2-inch pieces
1	tbsp. olive oil
¾	tsp. garlic-pepper blend (Lawry's)
2	large sweet onions, cut into 1-inch pieces
½	tsp. salt

Preheat oven to 425° F. Combine all ingredients in 13x9-inch baking dish, tossing to coat. Bake for 35 minutes or until tender, stirring occasionally.

Exchanges per ½-cup serving: 1½ breads, ½ fat

SOUTHERN CORNBREAD DRESSING

Serves 12

FOR THE CORNBREAD

1	tbsp. reduced-fat margarine
⅔	c. chopped onion
⅔	c. chopped celery
1	c. yellow cornmeal
1	c. all-purpose flour
½	tsp. salt
1	tbsp. baking powder
1 ¼	c. reduced-fat buttermilk
1	large egg, lightly beaten

Preheat oven to 425° F. Melt margarine in 9-inch cast iron skillet over medium heat. Sauté onion and celery for about 3 minutes. Combine cornmeal, flour, salt and baking powder in a large bowl. Add buttermilk, egg and onion mixture, stirring until just moist. Pour batter into skillet. Bake at 425° F for 25-30 minutes. Bake far enough ahead to let completely cool before making into dressing.

FOR THE DRESSING

1	recipe cornbread, cooled and crumbled
1	tsp. sage (optional)
½	tsp. black pepper
½	c. sliced green onions
4-5	c. low-salt chicken broth, heated
2	eggs, lightly beaten
	Vegetable cooking spray

Preheat oven to 400° F. Place crumbled cornbread in a large bowl. Stir in sage, pepper and green onions. Slowly add heated broth while stirring mixture with a spoon. Stir in beaten eggs. Spoon mixture into a 2-quart casserole dish coated with cooking spray. Bake uncovered at 400° F for 40-45 minutes.

Exchanges per 1½-cup serving: 2 breads, ½ fat

FRENCH-STYLE GREEN BEANS

Serves 12

6	c. green beans, cut into 2-in. pieces (about 1 pound)
1	tsp. olive oil
½	c. sliced green onions
4	garlic cloves, crushed
3	c. plum tomatoes, seeded and thinly sliced (about 1 pound)
2	tsp. dried leaf basil
¼	tsp. salt
¼	tsp. black pepper

Steam green beans for about 5 minutes or until tender. Heat oil in large saucepan and sauté onions and garlic for about a minute over medium heat. Add beans and sauté an additional 3 minutes. Add tomatoes and remaining ingredients; sauté for 2 more minutes.

Exchanges per ½-cup serving: ½ vegetable

BREAKFAST

1½	slices *Raisin French Toast*
1	tbsp. sugar-free syrup
1	c. grapefruit sections
1	c. nonfat milk

Exchanges: ½ meat, 2 breads, ½ fruit, 1 milk

CHRISTMAS MEAL

3	ozs. *Cinnamon-Apple Pork Tenderloin*
¾	c. *Orange-Glazed Sweet Potatoes*
1	c. green beans
2	c. mixed greens salad with 1 tbsp. light dressing
⅛	slice *Blue Ribbon Frozen Snickers Pie*

Exchanges: 3½ meats, 3½ breads, 2 vegetables, 1 fruit, 2½ fats

LUNCH OR DINNER

1	c. *Hearty Vegetable Soup*
2	c. large green salad with tomatoes, cucumbers, etc.
1	oz. turkey, cubed and placed on top of salad
1	tbsp. salad dressing (your choice = ½ fat)
3	crackers
1	c. yogurt with fresh fruit

Exchanges: 1 meat, 1 ½ breads, 2 vegetables, 1 ½ fruits, 1 milk, ½ fat

Total exchanges for day: 5 meats, 7 breads, 4 vegetables, 3 fruits, 2 milks, 3 fats

RAISIN FRENCH TOAST

Serves 1

¼	c. egg substitute
¼	tsp. vanilla flavoring
1	tsp. nonfat milk
1½	slices cinnamon-raisin bread
	Nonstick cooking spray

In a shallow bowl, combine egg substitute, vanilla and milk; add slices of bread, turning until egg mixture is absorbed. Spray a small nonstick skillet or griddle with nonstick cooking spray; preheat. Cook bread over medium heat 3 to 5 minutes, turning once, until golden brown on both sides.

Exchanges: ½ meat, 2 breads

CINNAMON-APPLE PORK TENDERLOIN

Serves 4

1	lb. pork tenderloin
2	apples, peeled, cored and sliced
2	tsp. cornstarch
1	tsp. ground cinnamon
2	tbsp. raisins

Preheat oven to 400° F. Place the tenderloin in roasting pan or casserole dish with a lid. In medium bowl, combine apples, cornstarch, cinnamon and raisins; stir. Spoon apple mixture around tenderloin. Cover and bake 40 minutes; remove lid and spoon mixture over top of tenderloin. Bake uncovered 15 to 20 minutes longer, or until tenderloin is browned and cooked through.

Exchanges per 3-oz. serving: 3 meats, 1 fruit

ORANGE-GLAZED SWEET POTATOES

Serves 4

3	c. sweet potatoes (about 2½ lbs.), peeled and thinly sliced
1	small lemon, thinly sliced
2	tsp. reduced-fat margarine
2⅔	tbsp. orange juice
1	tsp. grated orange rind

$3\frac{1}{2}$ tbsp. firmly packed brown sugar (or brown sugar substitute)
Nonstick cooking spray

Preheat oven to 400° F. Arrange potatoes and lemon slices in 13x9-inch baking dish coated with cooking spray; set aside. Melt margarine in small bowl. Add orange juice, orange rind and brown sugar to melted margarine; mix well to blend. Drizzle mixture over potatoes; cover dish with foil. Bake 35 minutes; uncover, stir and bake 30 minutes more.

Exchanges per $\frac{3}{4}$-cup serving: 2 breads, $\frac{1}{2}$ fat

~ ~

BLUE RIBBON FROZEN SNICKERS PIE

Serves 8

3	graham cracker squares
12	ozs. frozen vanilla yogurt or ice cream (fat-free, sugar-free)
1	c. Lite Cool Whip
3	tbsp. chunky peanut butter
1	1 oz. (4 serving size) box sugar-free chocolate pudding, dry

Crush graham crackers into fine crumbs and place in an 8x8-inch baking dish. Mix all other ingredients together. Pour into dish, being careful not to disturb crumbs. Freeze until firm. Remove from freezer 10 minutes before serving. Cut into 8 equal portions.

Exchanges per serving: $\frac{1}{2}$ meat, 1 bread, $\frac{1}{2}$ fat

~ ~

HEARTY VEGETABLE SOUP

Serves 10

1	bag frozen mixed vegetables
2	cans beef broth
1	can vegetable broth
1	can chicken broth
1	15-oz. can chopped tomatoes
4	medium potatoes, cut into bite-size pieces
$\frac{1}{2}$	lb. carrots, sliced
$\frac{1}{4}$	head cabbage, sliced
1	medium onion, chopped
	Basil and bay leaf to taste

Combine ingredients in a large pot. Simmer until vegetables are tender.

Exchanges: 1 bread, 2 vegetables

SPICED TEA MIX FOR GIFT GIVING

½	c. dry, plain instant tea
49	ozs. dry sugar-free lemonade-flavored Kool-Aid
1	can orange Crystal Light®, all 4 pkgs., dry
1	tbsp. ground cinnamon
1	tbsp. ground nutmeg

Mix all ingredients together. Divide into decorative jars or airtight containers with gift tag reading: "Use ¼ tsp. of spiced tea mix to 6 ounces water."
Exchanges per 6-oz. glass: Free

~~~~~~

CRANBERRY RELISH

Serves 4

1	thin-skinned orange, seeded and chopped
⅓	c. fresh cranberries
1	medium apple, unpeeled and chopped
1	8-oz. can unsweetened pineapple tidbits, drained

Position knife blade in food processor bowl; add orange. Cover with top; process 3 minutes or until orange peel is finely chopped. Add remaining ingredients and pulse 4 times, scraping sides of processor bowl between each pulse. Cover and chill.
Exchanges per ½-cup serving: 1 fruit

~~~~~~

SPICED FRUIT BUTTER

Makes six ½-pint jars

3	lbs. apples, pears or peaches
¾	c. apple juice, pear nectar or peach nectar
1 to 2	tsp. ground cinnamon
½	tsp. ground nutmeg
⅛	tsp. ground cloves
16	packets Equal® sweetener

Peel and core, or pit, fruit; slice. Combine prepared fruit, fruit juice and spices in Dutch oven. Bring to boil; cover and simmer until very tender, about 15 minutes. Cool slightly. Puree in batches in blender or food processor. Return to Dutch oven. Simmer, uncovered, over low heat until desired consistency, stirring frequently (this may take up to 1 hour.) Remove from heat; stir in Equal. Transfer to freezer containers or jars, leaving ½-inch headspace. Store up to 2 weeks in refrigerator or up to 3 months in freezer.

Exchanges per one tablespoon serving: Free

~~~~~~

MAPLE-GLAZED SWEET POTATOES

Serves 8

2	lbs. sweet potatoes, peeled, cut into 1-inch slices
1	c. frozen Granny Smith apple juice concentrate, thawed
2	tsp. cornstarch
7	packets Equal sweetener
1	tsp. margarine
1	tsp. maple extract
1	tsp. vanilla extract

Boil sweet potato slices until desired tenderness. Set aside and keep warm. Heat apple juice concentrate, cornstarch and Equal to boiling in small saucepan; boil, stirring constantly, until thickened. Remove from heat; stir in margarine, maple extract and vanilla extract. Pour glaze over potatoes in serving bowl and toss gently. Serve immediately.

Exchanges per serving: 1 bread

~~~~~~

PUMPKIN CHEESECAKE

Serves 8

3	3x6-inch graham cracker rectangles
2	8-oz. packages fat-free cream cheese
1	c. canned pumpkin
⅓	c. nonfat dry milk
1	4-oz. can evaporated skim milk
2	tsp. pumpkin pie spice
1	tsp. vanilla
1	1-oz. (4 servings) size package sugar-free vanilla instant pudding, dry
1	4-oz. Lite Cool Whip, thawed

Lay graham cracker rectangles in a 9x9-inch baking dish. In a bowl, cream together cream cheese, pumpkin, dry milk, canned milk, pumpkin pie spice and vanilla. Add the sugar-free pudding and mix thoroughly. Blend in Lite Cool Whip. Spread mixture evenly over graham crackers. Refrigerate for several hours before serving.

Exchanges per serving: 1 meat, 1½ breads, ¼ fat

~ ~

HOLIDAY FRENCH TOAST

Serves 2

2	tsp. blueberry sugar-free jelly or your favorite flavor
1	tsp. blueberry sugar-free jelly
4	slices diet bread
1	egg
1	egg white
2	tbsp. skim milk
2	ozs. fat-free cream cheese
	Nonstick cooking spray

In a small bowl, cream together cream cheese and 2 tsp. sugar-free jelly. Spread on the bread, making two sandwiches. Beat together egg, egg white and skim milk (Egg Beaters® or egg whites only may be substituted). Dip each sandwich in the mixture and coat each side. Place in a nonstick skillet sprayed with nonstick cooking spray and grill 3 minutes or until golden brown. Place remaining 1 tsp. of jelly in a small bowl with 1 tsp. of water and heat in a microwave oven until warm. Drizzle over French toast and serve immediately. **Optional:** Garnish with sliced peaches, bananas, or fruit of choice. (Be sure to count fruit exchanges, if garnish is added.)

Exchanges per serving: 1 meat, 1 bread, ¼ fat

~ ~

EASY CORNBREAD DRESSING

Serves 16

2	6-oz. packages cornbread mix
2	whole eggs
1⅓	c. skim milk
1½	c. chopped celery
1½	c. chopped onion
10	c. water
10	chicken bouillon cubes

1	tbsp. poultry seasoning
1	8-oz. package herb-seasoned cornbread stuffing mix
4	egg whites, beaten

Preheat oven to 375° F. Make cornbread according to package directions, using the 2 whole eggs and skim milk. Boil celery and onion in the water with the bouillon cubes over low heat for 3 to 5 minutes. Crumble cooked cornbread and combine with stuffing mix. Add poultry seasoning to boiled mixture and pour over bread mixture. After mixture has cooled, stir in beaten egg whites. Bake for 45 minutes.

Exchanges per ½ cup serving: 1½ breads, ½ fat

~~~~~~

GRAVY FOR CORNBREAD DRESSING

Serves 16

3	c. water
4	cubes chicken bouillon cubes
2	tbsp. flour
	Salt and pepper to taste

In a pan, bring water to boil. Add bouillon cubes. In a pint jar with lid, combine ¾ cup of the bouillon water with flour. Shake well. Pour this mixture into remaining water a little at a time to prevent lumps from forming. Cook over low heat, stirring frequently, until gravy consistency. May add more flour and water, if needed.

Exchanges per ¼ cup serving: Free

~~~~~~

CHOCOLATE CHEESECAKE

Serves 8

2	8-oz. packages fat-free cream cheese
1½	c. skim milk
2	packages sugar-free hot chocolate mix, dry
1	tsp. vanilla
1	3-oz. sugar-free chocolate pudding mix, dry
4	ozs. Lite Cool Whip
1	reduced-fat graham cracker pie crust

Cream softened cream cheese with ½ c. skim milk, using back of spoon. Add hot chocolate mix and vanilla. Beat remaining 1 c. milk with pudding mix.

Add to cream cheese mixture. Fold in Lite Cool Whip. Place in pie crust. Refrigerate several hours before serving.

Exchanges: 1 meat, 1 bread, ½ milk, ½ fat

~~~~~~

TURKEY SPAGHETTI

Serves 4

½	c. chopped onion
8	ozs. diced turkey
1	can low-fat cream of mushroom soup
4	oz. reduced-fat cheddar cheese, shredded
2	c. spaghetti noodles, cooked
1	small jar pimiento, chopped
1	tsp. dried parsley flakes
	Pepper, to taste
	Nonstick cooking spray

Preheat oven at 350° F. Spray large nonstick skillet with cooking spray. Sauté onion with turkey. Blend in mushroom soup and cheese. Cook over low heat until cheese is melted, stirring. Add cooked spaghetti, pimiento, parsley and pepper. Place mixture in a baking dish. Bake for 14 minutes.

Exchanges per ½ cup serving: 3 meats, 1 bread, ½ fat

~~~~~~

SINGLE-SERVING CHOCOLATE CAKE

Serves 1

1	pkg. instant sugar-free chocolate drink mix, dry
3	tbsp. flour
½	tsp. baking powder
2	packages artificial sweetener
1	tsp. vanilla
¼	c. water
1	tbsp. peanut butter
	Nonstick cooking spray

Preheat oven to 350° F. Mix dry ingredients together. Stir in vanilla and water. Add peanut butter. Spray individual-size loaf pan with nonstick cooking spray and pour batter into pan. Bake 15 minutes or until toothpick inserted in center comes out clean.

Exchanges per serving: 1 meat, 1 bread, 1 milk, 1 fat

PINEAPPLE CREAM CHEESE PIE

Serves 16

2	8-oz. packages fat-free cream cheese
¼	c. Equal Measure®
1	8-oz. Lite Cool Whip
1	tsp. vanilla
2	drops yellow food coloring
1	20-oz. can crushed pineapple in own juice, drained

Bring all ingredients to room temperature (about 1 hour). In a mixing bowl, cream the cream cheese and Equal Measure together; add the Lite Cool Whip and mix well. Add the remaining ingredients and mix well. Set aside.

FOR CRUMB CRUST

2	c. graham cracker crumbs
2	tbsp. Equal Measure®
4	tbsp. unsweetened applesauce

Combine all the ingredients. Press half of mixture in bottom of 10x12-inch pan. Pour cream cheese mixture over the crumb mixture. Sprinkle the remaining crumb mixture over the cream cheese mixture. Place in refrigerator for at least 4 hours to set.

Exchanges per serving: ½ meat, 1 bread, ½ fat

~~~~~~

RED HOLIDAY PUNCH

Serves 23

1	6-oz. package sugar-free cherry-flavored Jell-O
2	c. hot water
2	c. cold water
1	12-oz. can frozen orange juice concentrate, thawed
1	32-oz. can unsweetened pineapple juice
1	6-oz. can frozen pink sugar-free lemonade concentrate, thawed
1	tsp. vanilla
1	2-liter bottle Diet Sprite, Diet 7-UP or Diet Ginger Ale

Dissolve Jell-O in 2 cups hot water. Add 2 cups cold water and other ingredients. Chill. When ready to serve, add a 2-liter bottle of Diet Sprite, Diet 7-Up or Diet Ginger Ale.

Exchanges per 8-oz. serving: ½ fruit

SPINACH-PIMIENTO DIP

Serves 25

2	c. plain low-fat yogurt
¾	c. low-fat sour cream
5	ozs. chopped-frozen spinach, thawed
¼	c. green onions, minced
1	2-oz. jar pimiento, chopped
1	tbsp. Creole mustard
½	tbsp. Cavender's All-Purpose Green Seasoning (any all-purpose seasoning may be substituted)
½	tsp. garlic powder
	White pepper to taste
1	head of cabbage
	Fresh vegetables for dipping

In a medium bowl, whisk together yogurt and sour cream until smooth. Squeeze spinach to remove moisture. Stir spinach and remaining ingredients into the yogurt mixture. Chill for 1 to 2 hours before serving. Serve in a hollowed-out cabbage head with fresh vegetables arranged around the dip on a platter.

Exchanges per 1-cup serving vegetables: 1 vegetable; dip exchange is free

~~~~~~

SPINACH-ARTICHOKE DIP

Serves 12

1	9-oz. package frozen, no-salt-added artichoke hearts, thawed and drained
4	ozs. low-fat cream cheese, room temperature
1	10-oz. package frozen creamed spinach, thawed
½	c. plain nonfat yogurt
¼	c. thinly sliced green onions, green part only
1	tsp. salt-free Italian herb seasoning
⅛	tsp. salt

Thoroughly dry artichokes and chop into small pieces. In medium bowl, whisk together remaining ingredients, blending well. Stir in artichokes. Cover and refrigerate for at least 1 hour to allow flavors to blend. Stir before serving. Serve with toasted pita chips or sliced raw vegetables.

Exchanges for ¼ cup dip: ½ vegetable, ½ fat (Note: Count pita chips and/or raw vegetables exchanges separately.)

FRESH ASPARAGUS WITH TOASTED NUTS

Serves 4

1-1¼	lbs. fresh asparagus
1	c. water
2	tbsp. fresh lime juice
2	tbsp. diced pimiento
1	tbsp. toasted pine nuts or walnuts

Rinse asparagus and snap off tough ends. In a large skillet, bring water to a boil and add asparagus. Cover and steam asparagus until bright green, 2 to 3 minutes. Remove from heat, drain and arrange on a platter. Sprinkle with lime juice. Garnish with pimiento and pine nuts or walnuts. Serve warm or chilled.

Exchanges per ½-cup serving: 1 vegetable

~~~~~~

FRESH CRANBERRY AND WILD RICE PILAF

Serves 4

½	c. wild rice, uncooked
1	c. chicken broth
¼	c. raisins, dark or golden
5	scallions, chopped
½	c. chopped celery
1	tbsp. canola oil
1	c. fresh cranberries
1	tbsp. grated orange rind
½	tsp. dried thyme

Preheat oven to 350° F. Place wild rice, water and raisins in a saucepan and cook over medium heat for one hour, or until the rice is tender. Drain. Sauté the scallions and celery in the oil until tender. Add the cranberries, orange rind, thyme and rice. Place in an oven safe container, cover and bake at 350° F for 25 minutes. To use as stuffing, stuff two Cornish hens, a 3-lb. chicken, or use on the side with a turkey breast. Bake at 350° F for 1 hour.

Exchanges per ⅔-cup serving: 2 breads

~~~~~~

PUMPKIN CAKE

Serves 24

1	18.25-oz. low-fat yellow cake mix
¼	c. reduced-fat margarine, melted
1	egg, slightly beaten
1	30-oz. can pumpkin pie *mix*, with spices already added to pumpkin
2	eggs, beaten
⅔	c. evaporated skim milk
2	tbsp. sugar
1	tsp. cinnamon
	Nonstick cooking spray

Preheat oven to 350° F. Coat a 9x13-inch pan with cooking spray. Set aside ⅛ cup of cake mix. Mix margarine and one egg and add to remaining cake mix. Press slightly dry mixture into bottom of pan to form a crust. Combine pumpkin pie mix, two remaining eggs and evaporated skim milk. Pour over prepared crust. Mix the ⅛ cup reserved cake mix, sugar and cinnamon and sprinkle over pumpkin filling. Bake 45 to 55 minutes, or until filling is set.

Exchanges per serving: 1½ breads, 1 vegetable

~~~~~~

MARINATED CUCUMBERS

Serves 4

½	c. low-calorie Italian dressing
⅛	tsp. pepper
1	medium cucumber, peeled and thinly sliced
1	tbsp. diced pimientos
¼	c. thinly sliced radishes
2	tbsp. chopped fresh parsley

Combine Italian dressing and pepper in a medium bowl; stir well. Add cucumber, pimientos, radishes and parsley. Toss gently to coat. Cover and marinate in refrigerator for at least 4 hours.

Exchanges per serving: Free

~~~~~~

THREE-CHEESE TURKEY BAKE

Serves 10

8	oz. uncooked lasagna noodles
½	c. chopped onion

½	c. chopped green pepper
3	tbsp. diet margarine
1	10.75-oz. can low-fat cream of chicken soup
4	oz.-can sliced mushrooms, drained
½	c. chopped pimientos
⅓	c. nonfat milk
½	tbsp. dried basil, crushed
1	tbsp. chili powder
1½	c. low-fat cream-style cottage cheese
1½	c. shredded American cheese
½	c. grated parmesan cheese
2	c. cooked turkey or chicken

Preheat oven to 350° F. Cook lasagna noodles in boiling salted water, according to package directions. Drain well. Cook onion and green pepper in diet margarine until tender. Stir in soup, mushrooms, pimientos, milk, basil and chili powder. Lay half the noodles in a 13x9x2–inch dish; layer the noodles with half each of soup mixture, cottage cheese, American cheese and Parmesan cheese. Place remaining half of the noodles over cheeses, followed by sauce, cottage cheese and turkey or chicken. Bake for 45 minutes. Top with remaining American and parmesan cheeses and bake 2 minutes more, or until cheese melts.

Exchanges per serving: 2 meats, 1½ breads, ½ vegetable, 1 fat

~~~~~~

CHEX® PARTY MIX

Serves 16

¼	c. diet margarine
1	tbsp. Worcestershire sauce
¼	tsp. celery salt
¼	tsp. seasoned salt
¼	tsp. garlic salt
2	c. Chex rice cereal
2	c. Chex wheat cereal
2	c. Chex corn cereal
1	c. plain Cheerios®
1	c. pretzel sticks or oyster crackers
	Butter-flavored nonstick cooking spray

Preheat oven to 325° F. In a small saucepan, heat the butter and seasonings. In a very large bowl, toss the remaining ingredients with the butter mixture. Spray a large rectangular pan with 1-inch sides, with the cooking spray. Spread the cereal mixture evenly over the pan. Bake 20 minutes, stirring occasionally. Serve immediately or store in an airtight container. This makes a nice gift or an alternative to chips for brown bag lunches.

Exchanges per ½-cup serving: ½ bread, 1 fat

CHRISTMAS CORN

Serves 8

¼	c. chopped green bell pepper
½	c. chopped onion
2	c. frozen whole kernel corn
1	small jar chopped pimiento
¼	tsp. salt (optional)
¼	tsp. pepper
1	tsp. dried parsley
¼	c. fat-free French dressing
	Nonstick cooking spray

Sauté green pepper and onion in nonstick skillet sprayed with nonstick cooking spray. Stir in corn and add the other ingredients. Lower heat and cook for 5 minutes, stirring often.

Exchanges per ½-cup serving: 1 bread

BREAKFAST

1	slice whole-wheat toast
½	tbsp. light margarine
1	egg, poached
½	grapefruit
1	c. nonfat milk

Exchanges: 1 meat, 1 bread, 1 fruit, 1 milk, 1 fat

~~~~~~

NEW YEAR'S DAY MEAL

Black-Eyed Pea Soup

Southwestern Coleslaw

1   piece *Blue Ribbon Cornbread*

Creamy Fruit Salad

Exchanges: 2 meats, 2 breads, 1 vegetable, 1 fruit, 1 fat

~~~~~~

LUNCH OR DINNER

1	2-oz. slice *French Bread Vegetable Pizza*
1	c. raw mini carrots
¼	c. fat-free Ranch dressing (dip for carrots)

Exchanges: 2 meats, 2 breads, 1½ vegetables, 1 fat

~~~~~~

SNACKS

1	c. nonfat dairy yogurt with ½ banana (**Exchanges: 1 fruit, 1 milk**)
3	c. light microwave popcorn (**Exchanges: 1 bread**)
1	*Tortilla Roll-Up* (**Exchanges: 1 meat, 1 bread**)

~~~~~~

BLACK-EYED PEA SOUP

Serves 6

2	c. dried black-eyed peas (about 10 oz.)
2	tbsp. vegetable oil
1	large onion, chopped
1	tsp. minced garlic
1	c. chopped green bell pepper
5	c. canned fat-free chicken broth
1	bay leaf
1	tsp. salt
¼	tsp. dried red pepper flakes
12	ozs. diced smoked turkey
6	tsp. fat-free sour cream, optional
	Fresh cilantro sprigs for garnish, optional

Place the black-eyed peas in a large bowl and cover with cold water. Soak overnight. The next day, drain the peas, rinse thoroughly and drain again. In a large saucepan over medium-high heat, heat the oil. Sauté the onion and garlic in the oil until soft. Add the peas and the bell pepper, chicken stock, bay leaf, salt and red pepper flakes. Cover and bring to a boil. Reduce heat and simmer for 1 hour or until the peas are tender. Stir in the smoked turkey and simmer for another 15 minutes. Remove the bay leaf. Pour into serving bowls and top each serving with a teaspoon of sour cream and a sprig of cilantro, if desired.

Exchanges per 1-cup serving: 2 meats, 1 bread, 1 fat

SOUTHWESTERN COLESLAW

Serves 4

1	medium Savoy cabbage, untrimmed
½	c. coarsely shredded red cabbage
½	c. corn kernels
½	oz. low-fat cheddar cheese, shredded
⅓	c. chunky salsa
2	tbsp. plain nonfat yogurt

2	tsp. fat-free sour cream
¼	tsp. chili powder

Remove 4 leaves from the Savoy cabbage, set aside. Coarsely shred inner leaves; combine with red cabbage, corn and cheddar cheese in large bowl; set aside. In small bowl, combine salsa, yogurt, sour cream and chili powder; blend well. Add dressing to cabbage mixture, tossing gently. Cover and chill. Serve in reserved leaves.

Exchanges per 1-cup serving: 1 vegetable

~~~~~~

BLUE RIBBON CORNBREAD

Serves 12

1	c. cornmeal
1	c. all-purpose flour
½	tsp. salt
1	tbsp. baking powder
1	egg
1	c. nonfat milk
4	oz. artificially sweetened vanilla-flavored nonfat yogurt
	Nonstick cooking spray

Preheat oven to 425° F. In large bowl, combine cornmeal, flour, salt and baking powder; mix well. Add egg, milk and yogurt; stir to combine and pour into 9x9-inch baking dish coated with cooking spray. Bake 20 minutes.

Exchanges per serving: 1 bread

~~~~~~

CREAMY FRUIT SALAD

Serves 4

1	15-oz. can chunky mixed fruit in juice, drained
2	medium bananas, sliced
1	c. sliced strawberries
½	c. artificially sweetened lemon-flavored low-fat yogurt
½	c. fat-free whipped topping, thawed

Combine mixed fruit, bananas and strawberries in a medium bowl. Gently fold in yogurt and whipped topping until fruit is coated. Refrigerate until ready to serve.

Exchanges per 1-cup serving: 1 fruit

FRENCH BREAD VEGETABLE PIZZA

Serves 1

2	ozs. slice French bread
1½	tbsp. pizza sauce
2	ozs. part-skim mozzarella cheese
	Choice of onions, mushrooms, bell pepper or zucchini, sliced thin

Preheat oven to 375° F. Top bread with pizza sauce, cheese and vegetables. Bake until cheese melts, approximately 15 minutes.

Exchanges: 2 meats, 2 breads, ½ vegetable, 1 fat

~~~~~~

TORTILLA ROLL-UPS

Serves 6

6	6-in. low-fat flour tortillas
8	ozs. fat-free cream cheese
¼	c. chunky salsa

Mix cream cheese and salsa in small bowl; stir well to combine. Cover one side of each tortilla with an equal amount of cream-cheese blend; roll tortillas and place on serving platter. Cover with plastic wrap and refrigerate at least 1 hour. Slice into 1-inch pieces just prior to serving.

Exchanges per 1 roll-up: 1 meat, 1 bread

~~~~~~

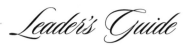

PURPOSE

- This First Place holiday session is six weeks in length with one meeting per week.
- The holiday session is recommended for those who have completed at least one regular session of First Place.
- The purpose of the holiday session is to provide accountability and encouragement for First Place members who desire to maintain their healthy habits through the holidays.

ONE-HOUR SESSION PLAN

15 minutes—Members weigh-in; Scripture memory verse

15 minutes—Holiday Helps spotlight

15 minutes—Devotional discussion

15 minutes—Prayer requests and prayer

WEEKLY ASSIGNMENTS

- Read a devotional daily and complete the journal section.
- Fill out a Commitment Record daily.
- Complete the assigned Holiday Helps Wellness Worksheet.

    Week 1—Holiday Goals

    Week 2—No-Worry Thanksgiving!

    Week 3—Holiday Survival Tips and Christmas Mission: Possible

    Week 4—Healthy Holiday Cooking Hints

    Week 5—Bring Joy to the Season

    Week 6—Emotional Traps

WEEK ONE

HOLIDAY GOALS WELLNESS WORKSHEET

Explain

Staying motivated during times like this can be difficult. But staying motivated can be difficult at any time of the year if we lose sight of how we benefit from our weight-loss efforts.

Discuss

1. Have you ever gained weight during the holidays?
2. What tempts you to overeat?
3. What's the payoff when you overeat? What do you get out of overeating?
4. What might you gain by staying focused during the holidays?

Guide the members to make realistic goals for the holiday session. Have them discuss in small groups or with the whole group some strategies that may keep them focused on their holiday goals. List these strategies on a whiteboard, chalkboard or poster board. Have them write down on the Wellness Worksheet the strategies they will try to implement during this holiday season.

GATES OF THANKSGIVING DISCUSSION

1. Invite volunteers to share about losses they have experienced and list any blessings that have come from the loss.
2. Ask members to share Scripture verses that have brought comfort or healing to their life.
3. Have members write on small index cards a praise or something for which they are thankful. Send a basket around and fill it with the blessings.
4. For the prayer time, read the praises, and then ask each member to pray by speaking a one-word praise (e.g., children, health, Jesus, etc.).

WEEK TWO

NO-WORRY THANKSGIVING! WELLNESS WORKSHEET

Explain

Anticipating challenges or obstacles faced on Thanksgiving will allow you time to develop strategies to overcome these challenges.

Discuss

1. Instruct members to write out what they plan to eat on Thanksgiving Day.

Refer them to the 1,400-calorie Thanksgiving Day menu and to the recipes that follow.

2. Ask members to share the strategies they are planning to use to overcome some of the challenges that this holiday will bring.

WONDERFUL WORKS DISCUSSION

1. Ask members to list the character traits of God. Then have volunteers explain how they have come to know more fully a specific character trait of God.
2. *Before the meeting,* write Psalm 139:14 on a whiteboard, chalkboard or poster board and display it in the room. Ask volunteers who have memorized the verse to quote it for the group. Then have each member tell one wonderful way God has created them (e.g., strong legs, excellent vision, a good singing voice).
3. Pray aloud using Psalm 139:14 as a prayer and then have volunteers pray and thank God for His wonderful works.

WEEK THREE

HOLIDAY SURVIVAL TIPS WELLNESS WORKSHEET

Explain

We all want to survive the holidays with our healthy habits still in place. Today, let's plan activities that will take us through the holidays and enable us to become healthier physically, emotionally, mentally and spiritually in the coming year.

Discuss

1. *Before the meeting,* call members and ask them to bring a calendar to the meeting. Using the Wellness Worksheet, ask them to select one activity that they would enjoy doing. Have them write that activity on a specific date of their calendar.
2. Ask them to list one activity for each of the four areas: physical, mental, emotional and spiritual.
3. Have members form pairs. Ask each partner to share what activity he or she plans to do that week, and then pray together about that activity.
4. Ask the members to check up on their partner that week and encourage that person to follow through with the activity he or she planned.

CHRISTMAS MISSION: POSSIBLE WELLNESS WORKSHEET

This Wellness Worksheet presents a Christmas-giving idea. Encourage members to invite their families or friends to participate in this mission as a way to place the focus on Christ and others during Christmas.

Birth of a Savior Discussion

1. **Before the meeting,** call a member and ask him or her to prepare to give a brief testimony of his or her salvation. Begin the meeting by inviting this member to share.
2. Ask members, "What is your focus during this holiday?" Invite volunteers to share how they as an individual or as a family, keep their focus on the birth of Christ rather than on buying gifts.
3. Discuss all of the roles that they take on, such as mom, dad, sister, wife, volunteer, Sunday School teacher, etc., during this busy season.
4. As a group, read Isaiah 9:6 aloud; then list the names of Jesus that are stated in this verse and ask members which name they need to call on to meet the needs of a specific responsibility that they must fulfill.

Note: For next week's meeting invite volunteers to bring in a holiday party food, such as a dip, finger food or treat, using one of the holiday recipes or one of their own light recipes. If they bring a recipe of their own, ask them to provide copies of the recipe for the other members. You may also want to make one of the holiday recipes as well. **Optional activity:** Have a recipe exchange. Invite members to bring copies of at least one light-eating recipe to share with others.

WEEK 4

Healthy Holiday Cooking Hints Wellness Worksheet

Explain

Today we will experiment with some healthy holiday recipes.

Discuss

1. Read through the Healthy Holiday Cooking Hints and ask members to share ideas for lightening up their favorite holiday recipes.
2. Discuss the 1,400-Calorie Christmas Day menu and recipes and how they plan on utilizing this tool.
3. **Option:** Have the "Recipe Exchange" and allow time for members to exchange their light holiday recipes while tasting the foods that were brought to class.

Gift of Love Discussion

1. Ask members to share with the group how God has shown His love to them specifically this week.
2. Brainstorm ways that they can show God's love to their neighbors or to the hard-to-love people in their lives.

3. Read Ephesians 3:16-19. Invite members to pray this Scripture for one another before closing in prayer.

WEEK 5

BRING JOY TO THE SEASON WELLNESS WORKSHEET

Explain

Today we will focus on spreading joy to others.

Activity

1. *Before the meeting,* gather blank cards and other supplies (construction paper, stickers, rubber stamps and stamp pads, felt-tip pens, glue, etc.) to make greeting cards. If you have a member who is crafty, enlist his or her help in showing members how to make a specific type of card, but keep it simple!

2. Have each member select one person whom they want to encourage. Have each member send that person a special New Year's card. Invite volunteers to share to whom they are sending the card and why.

3. Ask members to plan their New Year's Day menu, using the 1,400-calorie New Year's Day menus and recipes.

SPRING FORWARD DISCUSSION

1. Give each member a blank piece of paper and ask them to list anything in their past that they would consider a failure. Have them each silently ask God to forgive them for their part in the failure and then to ask God to make a way to correct this in their life and leave this incident in the past. After a few minutes of private prayer, have members tear up their paper and throw it in the trash (or even have a paper shredder handy for this task). This is a way of putting their failures in the past and forgetting them. **Option:** If you have a safe way to do this (i.e., a fireplace or outdoor barbeque or fire ring), invite members to burn the paper to signify that this is forgiven and forgotten by God.

2. Invite members to share the areas of commitment or situations in which they need God's power to accomplish a miracle. Pray Isaiah 48:14 that God would make a way through their specific situations.

3. Invite members to share their dreams for the new year by sharing what new thing they would like to accomplish.

WEEK 6

EMOTIONAL TRAPS WELLNESS WORKSHEET

Before the meeting, ask members to bring their calendars to class or make enough copies of a one-page yearly calendar for each member that will include the next few weeks. Bring multicolored felt-tip pens, yarn and scissors to class.

Explain

The holidays can be full of joy, but they can also bring many stresses to our lives. We must learn to manage these negative influences in our lives in order to maintain a healthy and balanced life.

Discuss

1. Have members form pairs and have them share holiday stressors. If they feel comfortable sharing, ask them to share if there are any special days or people that may cause them to be especially emotional. Have them pray for one another.
2. With the whole group using their calendars, have the members circle with a blue pen any day that they know will be emotionally difficult.
3. Have members give their name and the date(s) that will be hard; encourage the other members to put that member's name on that date so that they can remember to pray for him or her.
4. Instruct members to use a bright-colored pen, such as red or orange, to mark a star on those days that are party or celebration days.
5. Instruct members to select three days a week for exercise—a key to dealing with stress!—and circle those days with green pens.
6. Cut the yarn to make bracelets (or use a rubber band) to remind members to seek Christ first, not food, when an emotion becomes overwhelming. **Option:** You may even want to write something on a bracelet made of wide ribbon that will be a message of support, such as "Live strong—Seek the Son!"

NEW CREATION DISCUSSION

1. Invite members to share some old things that they need to get rid of this year: attitudes, habits, possessions, etc.
2. Explain that 2 Corinthians 5:17 suggests that we must "put on" the new self. Invite members to share which of the Nine Commitments they need to put on in the new year.
3. Have members brainstorm ways that they can support one another to remain faithful in keeping the commitments.
4. Challenge members to bring friends to the next orientation meeting to get the new year off to a great start!

COMMITMENT RECORDS

How to Fill Out a Commitment Record

The Commitment Record (CR) is an aid for you in keeping track of your accomplishments. Begin a new CR on the morning of the day your class meets. This ensures that your CR is complete before your next meeting. Turn in the CR weekly to your leader.

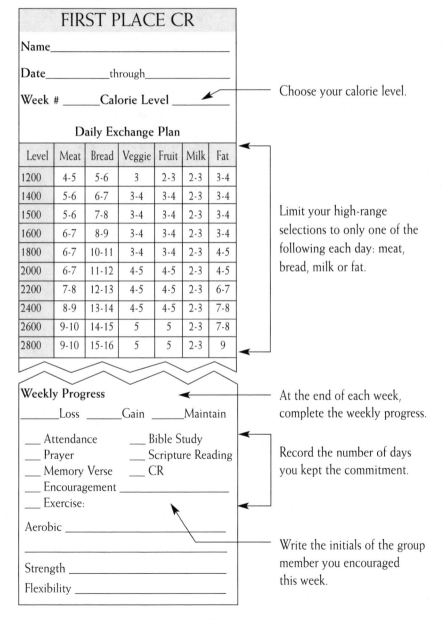

FIRST PLACE CR

Name_____

Date_____through_____

Week # _____Calorie Level _____

Choose your calorie level.

Daily Exchange Plan

Level	Meat	Bread	Veggie	Fruit	Milk	Fat
1200	4-5	5-6	3	2-3	2-3	3-4
1400	5-6	6-7	3-4	3-4	2-3	3-4
1500	5-6	7-8	3-4	3-4	2-3	3-4
1600	6-7	8-9	3-4	3-4	2-3	3-4
1800	6-7	10-11	3-4	3-4	2-3	4-5
2000	6-7	11-12	4-5	4-5	2-3	4-5
2200	7-8	12-13	4-5	4-5	2-3	6-7
2400	8-9	13-14	4-5	4-5	2-3	7-8
2600	9-10	14-15	5	5	2-3	7-8
2800	9-10	15-16	5	5	2-3	9

Limit your high-range selections to only one of the following each day: meat, bread, milk or fat.

Weekly Progress

_____Loss _____Gain _____Maintain

___ Attendance   ___ Bible Study
___ Prayer   ___ Scripture Reading
___ Memory Verse   ___ CR
___ Encouragement _____
___ Exercise:

Aerobic _____

_____

Strength _____

Flexibility _____

At the end of each week, complete the weekly progress.

Record the number of days you kept the commitment.

Write the initials of the group member you encouraged this week.

DAY 7: Date _____

Morning _____
_____
_____

Midday _____
_____
_____

Evening _____
_____
_____

Snacks _____
_____
_____

___ Meat _____   ☐ Prayer
___ Bread _____   ☐ Bible Study
___ Vegetable ____   ☐ Scripture Reading
___ Fruit _____   ☐ Memory Verse
___ Milk _____   ☐ Encouragement
___ Fat _____   ☐ Water_____

Exercise

Aerobic _____
_____

Strength _____

Flexibility _____

List the foods you have eaten. On this condensed CR it is not necessary to exchange each food choice. It will be the responsibility of each member that the tally marks you list below are accurate regarding each food choice. If you are unsure of an exchange, check the Live-It section of your copy of the *Member's Guide*.

List the daily food exchange choices to the left of the food groups.

Use tally marks for the actual food and water consumed.

Check off commitments completed. Use tally marks to record each 8-oz. serving of water.

List type and duration of exercise.

FIRST PLACE CR

Name _____

Date _____ through _____

Week # _____ Calorie Level _____

Daily Exchange Plan

Level	Meat	Bread	Veggie	Fruit	Milk	Fat
1200	4-5	5-6	3	2-3	2-3	3-4
1400	5-6	6-7	3-4	3-4	2-3	3-4
1500	5-6	7-8	3-4	3-4	2-3	3-4
1600	6-7	8-9	3-4	3-4	2-3	3-4
1800	6-7	10-11	3-4	3-4	2-3	4-5
2000	6-7	11-12	4-5	4-5	2-3	4-5
2200	7-8	12-13	4-5	4-5	2-3	6-7
2400	8-9	13-14	4-5	4-5	2-3	7-8
2600	9-10	14-15	5	5	2-3	7-8
2800	9-10	15-16	5	5	2-3	9

You may always choose the high range of vegetables and fruits. Limit your high range selections to only one of the following: meat, bread, milk or fat.

Weekly Progress

_____ Loss _____ Gain _____ Maintain

_____ Attendance _____ Bible Study
_____ Prayer _____ Scripture Reading
_____ Memory Verse _____ CR
_____ Encouragement:
_____ Exercise

Aerobic _____

Strength _____
Flexibility _____

DAY 7: Date _____

Morning _____

Midday _____

Evening _____

Snacks _____

_____ Meat ☐ Prayer
_____ Bread ☐ Bible Study
_____ Vegetable ☐ Scripture Reading
_____ Fruit ☐ Memory Verse
_____ Milk ☐ Encouragement
_____ Fat ☐ Water

Exercise
Aerobic _____

Strength _____
Flexibility _____

DAY 6: Date _____

Morning _____

Midday _____

Evening _____

Snacks _____

_____ Meat ☐ Prayer
_____ Bread ☐ Bible Study
_____ Vegetable ☐ Scripture Reading
_____ Fruit ☐ Memory Verse
_____ Milk ☐ Encouragement
_____ Fat ☐ Water

Exercise
Aerobic _____

Strength _____
Flexibility _____

DAY 5: Date _____

Morning _____

Midday _____

Evening _____

Snacks _____

_____ Meat ☐ Prayer
_____ Bread ☐ Bible Study
_____ Vegetable ☐ Scripture Reading
_____ Fruit ☐ Memory Verse
_____ Milk ☐ Encouragement
_____ Fat ☐ Water

Exercise
Aerobic _____

Strength _____
Flexibility _____

DAY 1: Date _____

Morning _____

Midday _____

Evening _____

Snacks _____

- ___ Meat   ☐ Prayer
- ___ Bread   ☐ Bible Study
- ___ Vegetable   ☐ Scripture Reading
- ___ Fruit   ☐ Memory Verse
- ___ Milk   ☐ Encouragement
- ___ Fat   ___ Water

Exercise
Aerobic _____
Strength _____
Flexibility _____

DAY 2: Date _____

Morning _____

Midday _____

Evening _____

Snacks _____

- ___ Meat   ☐ Prayer
- ___ Bread   ☐ Bible Study
- ___ Vegetable   ☐ Scripture Reading
- ___ Fruit   ☐ Memory Verse
- ___ Milk   ☐ Encouragement
- ___ Fat   ___ Water

Exercise
Aerobic _____
Strength _____
Flexibility _____

DAY 3: Date _____

Morning _____

Midday _____

Evening _____

Snacks _____

- ___ Meat   ☐ Prayer
- ___ Bread   ☐ Bible Study
- ___ Vegetable   ☐ Scripture Reading
- ___ Fruit   ☐ Memory Verse
- ___ Milk   ☐ Encouragement
- ___ Fat   ___ Water

Exercise
Aerobic _____
Strength _____
Flexibility _____

DAY 4: Date _____

Morning _____

Midday _____

Evening _____

Snacks _____

- ___ Meat   ☐ Prayer
- ___ Bread   ☐ Bible Study
- ___ Vegetable   ☐ Scripture Reading
- ___ Fruit   ☐ Memory Verse
- ___ Milk   ☐ Encouragement
- ___ Fat   ___ Water

Exercise
Aerobic _____
Strength _____
Flexibility _____

FIRST PLACE CR

Name _____

Date _____ through _____

Week # _____ Calorie Level _____

Daily Exchange Plan

Level	Meat	Bread	Veggie	Fruit	Milk	Fat
1200	4-5	5-6	3	2-3	2-3	3-4
1400	5-6	6-7	3-4	3-4	2-3	3-4
1500	5-6	7-8	3-4	3-4	2-3	3-4
1600	6-7	8-9	3-4	3-4	2-3	3-4
1800	6-7	10-11	3-4	3-4	2-3	4-5
2000	6-7	11-12	4-5	4-5	2-3	4-5
2200	7-8	12-13	4-5	4-5	2-3	6-7
2400	8-9	13-14	4-5	4-5	2-3	7-8
2600	9-10	14-15	5	5	2-3	7-8
2800	9-10	15-16	5	5	2-3	9

You may always choose the high range of vegetables and fruits. Limit your high range selections to only one of the following: meat, bread, milk or fat.

Weekly Progress

_____ Loss _____ Gain _____ Maintain

_____ Attendance _____ Bible Study
_____ Prayer _____ Scripture Reading
_____ Memory Verse _____ CR
_____ Encouragement:
_____ Exercise
Aerobic _____
Strength _____
Flexibility _____

DAY 5: Date _____

Morning _____

Midday _____

Evening _____

Snacks _____

_____ Meat   ☐ Prayer
_____ Bread   ☐ Bible Study
_____ Vegetable   ☐ Scripture Reading
_____ Fruit   ☐ Memory Verse
_____ Milk   ☐ Encouragement
_____ Fat   ☐ Water

Exercise
Aerobic _____
Strength _____
Flexibility _____

DAY 6: Date _____

Morning _____

Midday _____

Evening _____

Snacks _____

_____ Meat   ☐ Prayer
_____ Bread   ☐ Bible Study
_____ Vegetable   ☐ Scripture Reading
_____ Fruit   ☐ Memory Verse
_____ Milk   ☐ Encouragement
_____ Fat   ☐ Water

Exercise
Aerobic _____
Strength _____
Flexibility _____

DAY 7: Date _____

Morning _____

Midday _____

Evening _____

Snacks _____

_____ Meat   ☐ Prayer
_____ Bread   ☐ Bible Study
_____ Vegetable   ☐ Scripture Reading
_____ Fruit   ☐ Memory Verse
_____ Milk   ☐ Encouragement
_____ Fat   ☐ Water

Exercise
Aerobic _____
Strength _____
Flexibility _____

DAY 1: Date _____

Morning _____

Midday _____

Evening _____

Snacks _____

___ Meat ___	☐ Prayer
___ Bread ___	☐ Bible Study
___ Vegetable ___	☐ Scripture Reading
___ Fruit ___	☐ Memory Verse
___ Milk ___	☐ Encouragement
___ Fat ___	___ Water ___

Exercise
Aerobic _____
Strength _____
Flexibility _____

DAY 2: Date _____

Morning _____

Midday _____

Evening _____

Snacks _____

___ Meat ___	☐ Prayer
___ Bread ___	☐ Bible Study
___ Vegetable ___	☐ Scripture Reading
___ Fruit ___	☐ Memory Verse
___ Milk ___	☐ Encouragement
___ Fat ___	___ Water ___

Exercise
Aerobic _____
Strength _____
Flexibility _____

DAY 3: Date _____

Morning _____

Midday _____

Evening _____

Snacks _____

___ Meat ___	☐ Prayer
___ Bread ___	☐ Bible Study
___ Vegetable ___	☐ Scripture Reading
___ Fruit ___	☐ Memory Verse
___ Milk ___	☐ Encouragement
___ Fat ___	___ Water ___

Exercise
Aerobic _____
Strength _____
Flexibility _____

DAY 4: Date _____

Morning _____

Midday _____

Evening _____

Snacks _____

___ Meat ___	☐ Prayer
___ Bread ___	☐ Bible Study
___ Vegetable ___	☐ Scripture Reading
___ Fruit ___	☐ Memory Verse
___ Milk ___	☐ Encouragement
___ Fat ___	___ Water ___

Exercise
Aerobic _____
Strength _____
Flexibility _____

FIRST PLACE CR

Name _____

Date _____ through _____

Week # _____ Calorie Level _____

Daily Exchange Plan

Level	Meat	Bread	Veggie	Fruit	Milk	Fat
1200	4-5	5-6	3	2-3	2-3	3-4
1400	5-6	6-7	3-4	3-4	2-3	3-4
1500	5-6	7-8	3-4	3-4	2-3	3-4
1600	6-7	8-9	3-4	3-4	2-3	3-4
1800	6-7	10-11	3-4	3-4	2-3	4-5
2000	6-7	11-12	4-5	4-5	2-3	4-5
2200	7-8	12-13	4-5	4-5	2-3	6-7
2400	8-9	13-14	4-5	4-5	2-3	7-8
2600	9-10	14-15	5	5	2-3	7-8
2800	9-10	15-16	5	5	2-3	9

You may always choose the high range of vegetables and fruits. Limit your high range selections to only one of the following: meat, bread, milk or fat.

Weekly Progress

_____ Loss _____ Gain _____ Maintain

___ Attendance   ___ Bible Study
___ Prayer   ___ Scripture Reading
___ Memory Verse   ___ CR
___ Encouragement:
___ Exercise
Aerobic _____

Strength _____
Flexibility _____

DAY 5: Date _____

Morning _____

Midday _____

Evening _____

Snacks _____

___ Meat   ☐ Prayer
___ Bread   ☐ Bible Study
___ Vegetable ☐ Scripture Reading
___ Fruit   ☐ Memory Verse
___ Milk   ☐ Encouragement
___ Fat   Water _____

Exercise
Aerobic _____

Strength _____
Flexibility _____

DAY 6: Date _____

Morning _____

Midday _____

Evening _____

Snacks _____

___ Meat   ☐ Prayer
___ Bread   ☐ Bible Study
___ Vegetable ☐ Scripture Reading
___ Fruit   ☐ Memory Verse
___ Milk   ☐ Encouragement
___ Fat   Water _____

Exercise
Aerobic _____

Strength _____
Flexibility _____

DAY 7: Date _____

Morning _____

Midday _____

Evening _____

Snacks _____

___ Meat   ☐ Prayer
___ Bread   ☐ Bible Study
___ Vegetable ☐ Scripture Reading
___ Fruit   ☐ Memory Verse
___ Milk   ☐ Encouragement
___ Fat   Water _____

Exercise
Aerobic _____

Strength _____
Flexibility _____

Commitment Records 157

DAY 1: Date _____

Morning _____

Midday _____

Evening _____

Snacks _____

Food	Exercise
___ Meat	☐ Prayer
___ Bread	☐ Bible Study
___ Vegetable	☐ Scripture Reading
___ Fruit	☐ Memory Verse
___ Milk	☐ Encouragement
___ Fat ___ Water	

Exercise
Aerobic _____
Strength _____
Flexibility _____

DAY 2: Date _____

Morning _____

Midday _____

Evening _____

Snacks _____

Food	Exercise
___ Meat	☐ Prayer
___ Bread	☐ Bible Study
___ Vegetable	☐ Scripture Reading
___ Fruit	☐ Memory Verse
___ Milk	☐ Encouragement
___ Fat ___ Water	

Exercise
Aerobic _____
Strength _____
Flexibility _____

DAY 3: Date _____

Morning _____

Midday _____

Evening _____

Snacks _____

Food	Exercise
___ Meat	☐ Prayer
___ Bread	☐ Bible Study
___ Vegetable	☐ Scripture Reading
___ Fruit	☐ Memory Verse
___ Milk	☐ Encouragement
___ Fat ___ Water	

Exercise
Aerobic _____
Strength _____
Flexibility _____

DAY 4: Date _____

Morning _____

Midday _____

Evening _____

Snacks _____

Food	Exercise
___ Meat	☐ Prayer
___ Bread	☐ Bible Study
___ Vegetable	☐ Scripture Reading
___ Fruit	☐ Memory Verse
___ Milk	☐ Encouragement
___ Fat ___ Water	

Exercise
Aerobic _____
Strength _____
Flexibility _____

Name _____
Date _____ through _____
Week # _____ Calorie Level _____

Daily Exchange Plan

Level	Meat	Bread	Veggie	Fruit	Milk	Fat
1200	4-5	5-6	3	2-3	2-3	3-4
1400	5-6	6-7	3-4	3-4	2-3	3-4
1500	5-6	7-8	3-4	3-4	2-3	3-4
1600	6-7	8-9	3-4	3-4	2-3	3-4
1800	6-7	10-11	3-4	3-4	2-3	4-5
2000	6-7	11-12	4-5	4-5	2-3	4-5
2200	7-8	12-13	4-5	4-5	2-3	6-7
2400	8-9	13-14	4-5	4-5	2-3	7-8
2600	9-10	14-15	5	5	2-3	7-8
2800	9-10	15-16	5	5	2-3	9

You may always choose the high range of vegetables and fruits. Limit your high range selections to only one of the following: meat, bread, milk or fat.

Weekly Progress

_____ Loss _____ Gain _____ Maintain

_____ Attendance _____ Bible Study
_____ Prayer _____ Scripture Reading
_____ Memory Verse _____ CR
_____ Encouragement:
_____ Exercise
Aerobic _____

Strength _____
Flexibility _____

DAY 7: Date _____

Morning _____

Midday _____

Evening _____

Snacks _____

_____ Meat ☐ Prayer
_____ Bread ☐ Bible Study
_____ Vegetable ☐ Scripture Reading
_____ Fruit ☐ Memory Verse
_____ Milk ☐ Encouragement
_____ Fat ☐ Water

Exercise
Aerobic _____

Strength _____
Flexibility _____

DAY 6: Date _____

Morning _____

Midday _____

Evening _____

Snacks _____

_____ Meat ☐ Prayer
_____ Bread ☐ Bible Study
_____ Vegetable ☐ Scripture Reading
_____ Fruit ☐ Memory Verse
_____ Milk ☐ Encouragement
_____ Fat ☐ Water

Exercise
Aerobic _____

Strength _____
Flexibility _____

DAY 5: Date _____

Morning _____

Midday _____

Evening _____

Snacks _____

_____ Meat ☐ Prayer
_____ Bread ☐ Bible Study
_____ Vegetable ☐ Scripture Reading
_____ Fruit ☐ Memory Verse
_____ Milk ☐ Encouragement
_____ Fat ☐ Water

Exercise
Aerobic _____

Strength _____
Flexibility _____

DAY 1: Date _____

Morning _____

Midday _____

Evening _____

Snacks _____

___ Meat	☐ Prayer
___ Bread	☐ Bible Study
___ Vegetable	☐ Scripture Reading
___ Fruit	☐ Memory Verse
___ Milk	☐ Encouragement
___ Fat	___ Water

Exercise

Aerobic _____

Strength _____

Flexibility _____

DAY 2: Date _____

Morning _____

Midday _____

Evening _____

Snacks _____

___ Meat	☐ Prayer
___ Bread	☐ Bible Study
___ Vegetable	☐ Scripture Reading
___ Fruit	☐ Memory Verse
___ Milk	☐ Encouragement
___ Fat	___ Water

Exercise

Aerobic _____

Strength _____

Flexibility _____

DAY 3: Date _____

Morning _____

Midday _____

Evening _____

Snacks _____

___ Meat	☐ Prayer
___ Bread	☐ Bible Study
___ Vegetable	☐ Scripture Reading
___ Fruit	☐ Memory Verse
___ Milk	☐ Encouragement
___ Fat	___ Water

Exercise

Aerobic _____

Strength _____

Flexibility _____

DAY 4: Date _____

Morning _____

Midday _____

Evening _____

Snacks _____

___ Meat	☐ Prayer
___ Bread	☐ Bible Study
___ Vegetable	☐ Scripture Reading
___ Fruit	☐ Memory Verse
___ Milk	☐ Encouragement
___ Fat	___ Water

Exercise

Aerobic _____

Strength _____

Flexibility _____

FIRST PLACE CR

Name _____

Date _____ through _____

Week # _____ Calorie Level _____

Daily Exchange Plan

Level	Meat	Bread	Veggie	Fruit	Milk	Fat
1200	4-5	5-6	3	2-3	2-3	3-4
1400	5-6	6-7	3-4	3-4	2-3	3-4
1500	5-6	7-8	3-4	3-4	2-3	3-4
1600	6-7	8-9	3-4	3-4	2-3	3-4
1800	6-7	10-11	3-4	3-4	2-3	4-5
2000	6-7	11-12	4-5	4-5	2-3	4-5
2200	7-8	12-13	4-5	4-5	2-3	6-7
2400	8-9	13-14	4-5	4-5	2-3	7-8
2600	9-10	14-15	5	5	2-3	7-8
2800	9-10	15-16	5	5	2-3	9

You may always choose the high range of vegetables and fruits. Limit your high range selections to only one of the following: meat, bread, milk or fat.

Weekly Progress

Loss _____ Gain _____ Maintain

_____ Attendance _____ Bible Study
_____ Prayer _____ Scripture Reading
_____ Memory Verse _____ CR
_____ Encouragement:
_____ Exercise
Aerobic _____

Strength _____
Flexibility _____

DAY 5: Date _____

Morning _____

Midday _____

Evening _____

Snacks _____

_____ Meat   ☐ Prayer
_____ Bread   ☐ Bible Study
_____ Vegetable ☐ Scripture Reading
_____ Fruit   ☐ Memory Verse
_____ Milk   ☐ Encouragement
_____ Fat   _____ Water

Exercise
Aerobic _____

Strength _____
Flexibility _____

DAY 6: Date _____

Morning _____

Midday _____

Evening _____

Snacks _____

_____ Meat   ☐ Prayer
_____ Bread   ☐ Bible Study
_____ Vegetable ☐ Scripture Reading
_____ Fruit   ☐ Memory Verse
_____ Milk   ☐ Encouragement
_____ Fat   _____ Water

Exercise
Aerobic _____

Strength _____
Flexibility _____

DAY 7: Date _____

Morning _____

Midday _____

Evening _____

Snacks _____

_____ Meat   ☐ Prayer
_____ Bread   ☐ Bible Study
_____ Vegetable ☐ Scripture Reading
_____ Fruit   ☐ Memory Verse
_____ Milk   ☐ Encouragement
_____ Fat   _____ Water

Exercise
Aerobic _____

Strength _____
Flexibility _____

DAY 1: Date _____

Morning _____

Midday _____

Evening _____

Snacks _____

☐ Prayer
☐ Bible Study
☐ Scripture Reading
☐ Memory Verse
☐ Encouragement

Meat _____
Bread _____
Vegetable _____
Fruit _____
Milk _____
Fat _____
Water _____

Exercise
Aerobic _____
Strength _____
Flexibility _____

DAY 2: Date _____

Morning _____

Midday _____

Evening _____

Snacks _____

☐ Prayer
☐ Bible Study
☐ Scripture Reading
☐ Memory Verse
☐ Encouragement

Meat _____
Bread _____
Vegetable _____
Fruit _____
Milk _____
Fat _____
Water _____

Exercise
Aerobic _____
Strength _____
Flexibility _____

DAY 3: Date _____

Morning _____

Midday _____

Evening _____

Snacks _____

☐ Prayer
☐ Bible Study
☐ Scripture Reading
☐ Memory Verse
☐ Encouragement

Meat _____
Bread _____
Vegetable _____
Fruit _____
Milk _____
Fat _____
Water _____

Exercise
Aerobic _____
Strength _____
Flexibility _____

DAY 4: Date _____

Morning _____

Midday _____

Evening _____

Snacks _____

☐ Prayer
☐ Bible Study
☐ Scripture Reading
☐ Memory Verse
☐ Encouragement

Meat _____
Bread _____
Vegetable _____
Fruit _____
Milk _____
Fat _____
Water _____

Exercise
Aerobic _____
Strength _____
Flexibility _____

FIRST PLACE CR

Name _____

Date _____ through _____

Week # _____ Calorie Level _____

Daily Exchange Plan

Level	Meat	Bread	Veggie	Fruit	Milk	Fat
1200	4-5	5-6	3	2-3	2-3	3-4
1400	5-6	6-7	3-4	3-4	2-3	3-4
1500	5-6	7-8	3-4	3-4	2-3	3-4
1600	6-7	8-9	3-4	3-4	2-3	3-4
1800	6-7	10-11	3-4	3-4	2-3	4-5
2000	6-7	11-12	4-5	4-5	2-3	4-5
2200	7-8	12-13	4-5	4-5	2-3	6-7
2400	8-9	13-14	4-5	4-5	2-3	7-8
2600	9-10	14-15	5	5	2-3	7-8
2800	9-10	15-16	5	5	2-3	9

You may always choose the high range of vegetables and fruits. Limit your high range selections to only one of the following: meat, bread, milk or fat.

Weekly Progress

_____ Loss _____ Gain _____ Maintain

_____ Attendance _____ Bible Study
_____ Prayer _____ Scripture Reading
_____ Memory Verse _____ CR
_____ Encouragement:
_____ Exercise

_____ Aerobic _____

Strength _____
Flexibility _____

DAY 7: Date _____

Morning _____

Midday _____

Evening _____

Snacks _____

☐ Prayer — Meat
☐ Bible Study — Bread
☐ Scripture Reading — Vegetable
☐ Memory Verse — Fruit
☐ Encouragement — Milk
☐ Water — Fat

Exercise
Aerobic _____

Strength _____
Flexibility _____

DAY 6: Date _____

Morning _____

Midday _____

Evening _____

Snacks _____

☐ Prayer — Meat
☐ Bible Study — Bread
☐ Scripture Reading — Vegetable
☐ Memory Verse — Fruit
☐ Encouragement — Milk
☐ Water — Fat

Exercise
Aerobic _____

Strength _____
Flexibility _____

DAY 5: Date _____

Morning _____

Midday _____

Evening _____

Snacks _____

☐ Prayer — Meat
☐ Bible Study — Bread
☐ Scripture Reading — Vegetable
☐ Memory Verse — Fruit
☐ Encouragement — Milk
☐ Water — Fat

Exercise
Aerobic _____

Strength _____
Flexibility _____

DAY 1: Date _____

Morning _____

Midday _____

Evening _____

Snacks _____

___ Meat ___   ☐ Prayer
___ Bread ___   ☐ Bible Study
___ Vegetable ___   ☐ Scripture Reading
___ Fruit ___   ☐ Memory Verse
___ Milk ___   ☐ Encouragement
___ Fat ___   ___ Water ___

Exercise
Aerobic _____
Strength _____
Flexibility _____

DAY 2: Date _____

Morning _____

Midday _____

Evening _____

Snacks _____

___ Meat ___   ☐ Prayer
___ Bread ___   ☐ Bible Study
___ Vegetable ___   ☐ Scripture Reading
___ Fruit ___   ☐ Memory Verse
___ Milk ___   ☐ Encouragement
___ Fat ___   ___ Water ___

Exercise
Aerobic _____
Strength _____
Flexibility _____

DAY 3: Date _____

Morning _____

Midday _____

Evening _____

Snacks _____

___ Meat ___   ☐ Prayer
___ Bread ___   ☐ Bible Study
___ Vegetable ___   ☐ Scripture Reading
___ Fruit ___   ☐ Memory Verse
___ Milk ___   ☐ Encouragement
___ Fat ___   ___ Water ___

Exercise
Aerobic _____
Strength _____
Flexibility _____

DAY 4: Date _____

Morning _____

Midday _____

Evening _____

Snacks _____

___ Meat ___   ☐ Prayer
___ Bread ___   ☐ Bible Study
___ Vegetable ___   ☐ Scripture Reading
___ Fruit ___   ☐ Memory Verse
___ Milk ___   ☐ Encouragement
___ Fat ___   ___ Water ___

Exercise
Aerobic _____
Strength _____
Flexibility _____

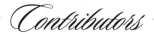

Carole Lewis, National Director of First Place, is a popular speaker and author of the books *Choosing to Change, First Place, Today Is the First Day, Back on Track, The Mother-Daughter Legacy* and *The Divine Diet*. Carole regularly leads conferences, F.O.C.U.S. weeks and seminars across the country. Her audiences know her as warm, transparent, honest and humorous.

Beverly Henson is a First Place networking leader in Mississippi, a certified personal trainer and a Bible teacher. Beverly speaks at First Place conferences and rallies and writes a monthly article on fitness for the First Place e-newsletter. Beverly has a genuine love of proclaiming the Word of God to His people.

Kay Smith is the Associate National Director of First Place. Having served on staff at First Baptist Church—the birthplace of the First Place program—in Houston, Texas, since 1987, Kay is also a popular speaker at retreats, seminars, conferences, F.O.C.U.S. weeks and workshops across the country. Her delightful personality and love for people endears her to everyone she meets. Kay and her husband, Joe, live in Roscoe, Texas, and have two children and five grandchildren.

Pat Lewis is Carole Lewis's assistant and First Place office manager. She was a member of the original First Place class in 1981 and assists Carole in leading First Place groups at Houston's First Baptist Church. Pat was also a contributing writer to the *Today Is the First Day* devotional book.

Nancy Taylor, First Place LeadershipTraining Director, teaches leadership principles to First Place leaders throughout the country and writes a monthly article for the First Place e-newsletter. She delights her audiences with humor and encourages them with boldness. Nancy was also a contributor to *Today Is the First Day*.

Stephanie Cheves was a staff member at First Place for many years and a faithful First Place leader at Houston's First Baptist Church. Stephanie has been blessed to work for and serve under some very godly individuals who have encouraged her in her faith throughout her career. Stephanie was also a contributor to *Today Is the First Day*. Stephanie and her husband, Chris, live in Houston, Texas, with their dog, Penny.

Scott Wilson, C.E.C., A.A.C., has been cooking professionally for 25 years. A certified executive chef with the American Culinary Federation, he currently works in the Greater Atlanta area as a personal chef and food consultant and is a Certified Personal Chef with the United States Personal Chef Association. Along with serving as the national food consultant for First Place, he is on the culinary program advisory board of the Art Institute in Atlanta. Scott has authored two cookbooks, *Dining Under the Magnolia* and *Healthy Home Cooking*. He is active in church work and enjoys spending time with his wife, Jennifer, and their daughter, Katie.

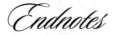

WEEK ONE

1. Jana Drake, "Can I Trust You Lord?" © 1988, *In the Cradle of Your Love* (Houston, TX: Ambient Productions, 1996).

WEEK TWO

1. Dr. Dick Couey, *Building God's Temple* (Edina, MN: Burgess International Group, Inc. 1987), p. 1.
2. Noah Webster, *Noah Webster's 1828 American Dictionary of the English Language* (San Francisco: Foundation for American Christian Education, 1967), s.v. "Thanksgiving Day."

WEEK FOUR

1. Zig Ziglar, *See You at the Top* (New York: Pelican Publishing Company, 1975), p. 288.

Biblically Based Reading
for Healthy Living

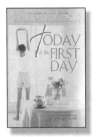

Today Is the First Day
Daily Encouragement on the Journey to
Weight Loss and a Balanced Life
Carole Lewis, General Editor
ISBN 08307.30656

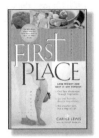

First Place
Lose Weight and Keep It Off Forever
Carole Lewis
ISBN 08307.28635

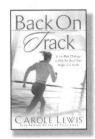

Back on Track
A 16-Week Challenge to Help You
Reach Your Weight-Loss Goals
Carole Lewis
ISBN 08307.32586

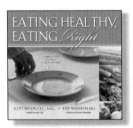

**Eating Healthy,
Eating Right**
A Complete 16-Week Meal Planner
to Help You Lose Weight
Scott Wilson, C.E.C., A.A.C.
and *Jody Wilkinson*, M.D.
ISBN 08307.30222

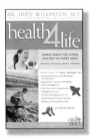

Health 4 Life
55 Simple Ideas for Living
Healthy in Every Area
Jody Wilkinson, M.D.
ISBN 08307.30516

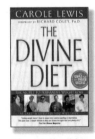

First Place Favorites
Favorite Recipes from the Nation's #1
Christian Weight-Loss Program
Carole Lewis, General Editor
ISBN 08307.32314

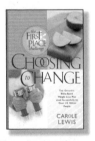

Choosing to Change
The Bible-Based Weight Loss Plan Used
Successfully by Over a Half Million People
Carole Lewis
ISBN 08307.28627

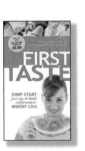

First Taste
Jump-Start Your Way to Health and
Permanent Weight Loss
ISBN 08307.38096

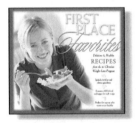

The Divine Diet
The Secret to Permanent Weight Loss
ISBN 08307.36271

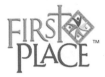

Available at bookstores everywhere or by calling
1-800-4-GOSPEL. **Join the First Place community
and order products at www.firstplace.org.**

Gospel Light